EASY EXERCISES FOR

STRENGTH & POWER

The Stay Fit Series

A Special Report published
by the editors of *Healthy Years*
in conjunction with
the David Geffen School of Medicine at UCLA
Division of Geriatrics

Easy Exercises for Strength & Power

Consulting Editor, Ellen Wilson, PT, Director of Therapy Services, UCLA Health

Author, Jim Brown, PhD, Executive Editor, Steadman Philippon Research Institute
Group Directors, Belvoir Media Group: Diane Muhlfeld, Jay Roland
Creative Director, Belvoir Media Group: Judi Crouse
Belvoir Editor: Matthew Solan
Illustrator: Alayna Paquette

Publisher, Belvoir Media Group: Timothy H. Cole

ISBN 978-1-879620-31-5

To order additional copies of this report or for customer service questions, please call 877-300-0253, or write to Health Special Reports, 535 Connecticut Avenue, Norwalk, CT 06854

RECENT FINDINGS

- Lower back pain top cause of disability (Page 8, Box 1-2).

- Resistance training increases leg strength in older adults (Page 10, Box 1-4).

- Endurance and resistance exercise lowers systolic and diastolic blood pressure (Page 10, Box 1-5).

- Resistance training and dietary changes prevent loss of lean body mass (Page 12, Box 1-8).

- Resistance training effective in reducing the risk of type 2 diabetes (Page 13, Box 1-9).

- Older adults in the best physical condition have the best mental abilities (Page 14, Box 1-10).

- Most effective peer pressure to improve fitness may come from spouse (Page 16, Box 1-12).

- Daily routines, positive feelings make adherence to exercise more likely (Page 17, Box 1-13).

- Increasing the velocity of power training could make older adults safer (Page 19, Box 1-15).

- Combined endurance and strength training improves muscle quality in older adults (Page 20, Box 1-16).

- Order of strength and aerobic training has no effect on performance or recovery (Page 21, Box 1-18).

- Chair-based exercises enhance strength and flexibility in older adults (Page 28, Box 2-9).

- Twenty-one million Americans have done yoga during the past year (Page 29, Box 2-11).

- The shoulder is a common injury site in resistance training (Page 38, Box 2-16).

Easy Exercises for
Strength & Power

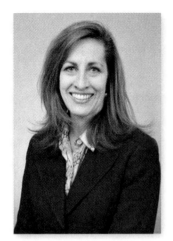

Ellen G. Wilson, PT
Director of Therapy Services
UCLA Health

A Message from the David Geffen School of Medicine at UCLA and Ellen Wilson, PT, Director of Therapy Services, UCLA Health

IF you are ready for an exercise program to maintain strength, or even get stronger with age, we think *Easy Exercises for Strength & Power* is the place to begin.

This Special Report is the fifth in the UCLA's Stay Fit Series, following *Balance & Mobility, Core Fitness, Aerobic Fitness*, and *Flexibility*.

Easy Exercises for Strength & Power has all the information you need to begin a program today. There are 40 exercises for the upper body, core, and lower body with step-by-step instructions and illustrations. Each one is age-appropriate and designed so you can get stronger at your own pace.

You can design your own program, or use one of the 11 strength and power exercise programs, including those for entry-level, intermediate, and advanced exercisers.

In addition, *Strength & Power* keeps you up-to-date with "Recent Findings" and exercise practices recommended by physicians, researchers, and physical therapists at UCLA and other major teaching institutions around the world.

To plan your exercise sessions and record your progress, there are copy-ready checklists and daily and weekly workout logs and calendars.

We at UCLA want you to be fit and that includes being strong enough to enjoy the activities of daily life with friends and family. Many of you have already begun your fitness program using previous reports in the Stay Fit Series. We hope *Easy Exercises for Strength & Power* will be just as helpful. As always, we're ready to help when you're ready.

Table of Contents

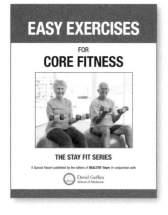

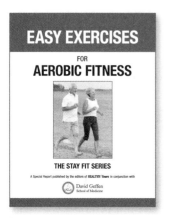

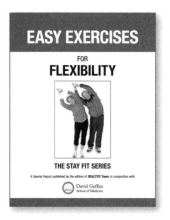

Easy Exercises for
Strength & Power

A preview

Chapter 1, *Strength & Power Training Decision,* takes you beyond the obvious advantages of maintaining strength to get through daily activities. It explains the importance of strength for conditions as diverse as arthritis and diabetes, back pain, blood pressure and bone health, and even emotional health. You also get an account of what a strength-training program costs in terms of money, time, and effort.

▶ Chapter 2, *Before You Begin*, begins with three easy self-tests to determine your own strength, then tells you about resistance training equipment, alternative ways to exercise, what to wear, what to eat, and how to recognize, prevent, and treat injuries associated with exercising to get stronger.

▶ Chapter 3, *40 Strength & Power Exercises,* is the heart of this Special Report. It describes and illustrates exercises you can learn to do at home using your own body weight as resistance, or inexpensive equipment, such as dumbbells, resistance bands, and medicine balls. And if you are uncertain about your ability to do any of the exercises, Chapter 3 suggests 14 ways to modify the exercises to fit your needs and fitness level.

▶ Chapter 4, *Strength & Power Exercise Programs,* has 11 pre-packaged programs from which you can choose to begin or continue a resistance routine. It includes two entry-level routines, followed by two packages for intermediates and two for advanced-level exercisers. And there are two chair-based packages for those who may not be mobile enough (yet) to perform exercises that require standing as well as routines the revolve around specific equipment like medicine and stability balls and resistance bands.

▶ Chapter 5, *The Strength & Power Workbook*, follows the format of the previous reports in the Stay Fit Series, and gives you the tools to schedule and monitor your progress. The *Daily Strength & Power Exercise Log* is a daily record-keeping cut-out for you to scan or copy so you can record each exercise performed, including the number of repetitions and sets. The *Two-Week Workout* outlines a sample two-week schedule that combines strength training with cross-training activities, like aerobic, balance, and flexibility, to create a well-rounded fitness program.

▶ Appendix I, *Glossary*. What's the difference between strength and power? Dumbbell and barbell? Check the *Glossary* for definitions of 67 strength, power, and fitness-related terms.

▶ Appendix II, *Resources*. Need more information? *Resources* has contact information for 20 health and fitness-related organizations.

1 STRENGTH & POWER TRAINING DECISION

D ecades of scientific evidence have made clear two important health and fitness issues: 1) At some point—probably in our mid-30s—we begin to lose muscle mass, muscle strength, and muscle function if we don't engage in a program of strength training that involves all of the body's major muscle groups. 2) It is *never* too late to begin and benefit from a strength (resistance) training program.

Those two facts mean we must make a decision regarding one of the oldest clichés in medical history: "Use it or lose it." If we take the "use it" option, we will begin to see results in a matter of weeks. With continued strength and power-based activities, the benefits will last a lifetime.

If we choose the "lose it" option (not doing anything about the inevitable loss of muscle size and strength), there is little good to expect from the consequences of that decision.

This Special Report makes the case for strength training within the context of a total fitness program. It encourages you to choose the "use it" option, and it gives you the tools to help you achieve your strength and fitness goals.

Total fitness includes aerobic capacity, balance, mobility, flexibility, and strength. Without strength as a foundation, the other fitness advantages are difficult to achieve.

When we say "strength training" what exactly does that mean? Strength training—also referred to as resistance training—is any exercise that uses some form of resistance to strengthen and build muscle. You create that resistance, and put your muscles to work, by using weight machines, dumbbells, resistance bands, stability and medicine balls, and even your own body weight.

But for many middle-aged and older adults, strength training evokes images of young athletes lifting heavy barbells in a sweaty, noisy gym. It is no surprise then that most adults resist strength training.

A study published in the *Journal of Strength and Conditioning Research* found that only 21 percent of adults participated in strength-training activities at least two days a week. The likelihood of participating was lower among older adults and women.

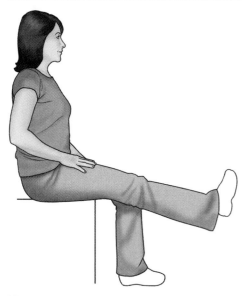

Knee extensions are an example of strength training and have been proven to increase strength and reduce pain caused by osteoarthritis.

Lower back pain top cause of disability

An international team of researchers designed a study to estimate the global burden of 291 conditions, including low back pain. Low back pain was identified as pain at any point from the lower margin of the ribs to the gluteal muscles (buttocks). The group gathered data on prevalence, incidence, remission, and duration. Lower back pain ranked highest in disability and sixth in overall burden, and the number of people around the world with the condition is expected to rise with aging populations in developed countries.

Annals of the Rheumatic Diseases, March 2014

Benefits beyond strength

Maintaining or improving strength just to get stronger is a worthy goal in itself, but strength has added value. Strong muscles and muscle groups affect almost every system of the body, every physical activity of daily living, and help combat many common health conditions.

Arthritis

Researchers at Tufts University found that older men and women with knee osteoarthritis (OA) who participated in a 16-week strength-training program had a 43 percent decrease in pain. The subjects also reported increased muscle strength, better overall physical performance, decreased disability, and improved symptoms of the condition.

Clinics in Geriatric Medicine published a review of multiple studies and concluded that progressive resistance training by older people with OA produced lower extremity strength and function, as well as pain reduction.

In the *Journal of Orthopaedic & Sports Physical Therapy*, research teams from UCLA and the National Taiwan University found that non-weight bearing strength training resulted in an increase in knee extensor muscle strength. (See Box 1-1, "Knee Extensions" for an example.)

"Strengthening exercises help maintain and improve your muscle strength. Strong muscles can support and protect joints that are affected by arthritis," says The Arthritis Foundation.

Back pain

Eighty-five percent of Americans will have lower back pain at some point in their lives. It is the second most common reason for seeing a physician. For 90 percent of the population, lower back pain often resolves within two to four weeks, with rest. But the rate of recurrence can be as high as 80 percent.

In fact, a study in a recent issue of *Annals of the Rheumatic Diseases* suggests that lower back pain causes more disability worldwide than any other condition (see Box 1-2, "Lower back pain top cause of disability"). With the number of older adults in the U.S. increasing rapidly, the incidence of low back pain is also likely to increase.

Strength training can help with recovery and even prevention. The main cause of low back pain is weak core muscles—those in the hips, pelvis, abdomen, and trunk. The core has to be strong to support your body's weight. When excessive pressure is put on the structures that form the spinal column, pain can be severe and serious injury is a possibility.

Muscle weakness doesn't necessarily mean that a person always feels weak in the core area, but rather in the arms and legs. A strong core transfers strength and provides power that allows for quick, strong, and efficient movement needed to lift, push, pull, and walk.

Weak core muscles get stronger with a strength training program that focuses on specific core muscle groups. Fifty core strength exercises are described in the Stay Fit Series report, *Easy Exercises for Core Fitness*.

Balance

Strength in the arms, legs, and core muscles provides the foundation for good balance. If you have trouble pushing with your arms to get out of a chair or off the sofa, it may be a sign of upper body weakness. If you are at times unsteady on your feet, the cause could be weakness in the lower part of the core or in your leg muscles. It could also be a warning that you are at higher risk for falls and decreased mobility.

The four-part quadriceps, as well as the muscles of the buttocks and hip, are particularly important for balance and stability. These muscles can keep you from stumbling when you trip on a rug or other objects, and from losing your balance when there is a change in momentum, which can happen when you are standing on a bus or train. The quads help stabilize the knee joint and reduce stress on knees affected by osteoarthritis. "Step-ups," illustrated in Box 1-3, are good for the muscles of the upper and lower legs and hips.

Three studies over the past five years reflect the body of evidence supporting strength training for better balance and improved mobility. For instance:

- Adults age 50 to 75 with diabetes had impaired balance, slow reaction time, and a higher risk for falls, but all three variables improved after resistance and balance training. —*Diabetes Care*, April 2010
- Australian researchers found that a program integrating principles of balance and strength training into everyday activities resulted in significant improvements in strength, function, and participation in habitual physical activity. —*BMJ*, June 2012
- In Germany and England, a research team reported that resistance and balance training increased leg strength in older

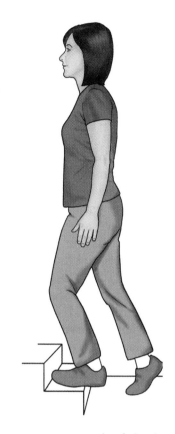

Step-ups are an example of simple, yet effective, quad-strengthening exercise you can do at home.

Resistance training increases leg strength in older adults

Researchers in Germany and England addressed the issue of decreasing maximal force produced during leg muscle contraction among people over the age of 65. They designed a program that compared leg strength differences between younger and older adults, then measured the effects of a resistance-training program and compared the results to balance-only training in both groups. They concluded that both programs improved strength and balance, and that the older adults increased leg strength almost to the level of their younger counterparts.

PLOS, February 19, 2015

Endurance and resistance exercise lowers systolic and diastolic blood pressure

Scientists in Belgium and Australia conducted a meta-analysis on the effects of various types of exercise on resting blood pressure in adults. The authors reviewed 93 trials involving more than 5,000 participants. They concluded that endurance training, dynamic resistance training (in which muscle and muscle groups move against resistance throughout an exercise), and isometric resistance training (in which the muscles do not move) all lower systolic and diastolic blood pressure. Data from a small number of isometric resistance training studies suggest that this form of exercise has potential for the greatest reduction in blood pressure.

Journal of the American Heart Association, February 1, 2013

adults. —*PLOS,* February 19, 2015 (see Box 1-4, "Resistance training increases leg strength in older adults").

Blood pressure

The American Heart Association is on record as supporting physical activity, including well-rounded strength training, to help lower blood pressure.

In one of the largest analyses of the effects of exercise training on blood pressure to date, the *Journal of the American Heart Association* said that endurance and resistance training lowers both systolic (top number) and diastolic (bottom number) blood pressure (see Box 1-5, "Endurance and resistance exercise lowers systolic and diastolic blood pressure").

However, the Mayo Clinic warns that one form of strength training—weight lifting—is not appropriate for everyone. Weight lifting is a type of strength training that uses free weights for resistance. "You shouldn't lift weights if your blood pressure is uncontrolled, meaning it is higher than 180/100 mmHg. If your blood pressure is higher than 160/100 mmHg, check with your doctor before beginning a weight-lifting program," according to the Mayo Clinic.

This advice is consistent with the suggestion that before beginning any new exercise program, you should ask for medical clearance from your family physician or other healthcare provider.

Bone health

Strength training rebuilds muscle mass, strength, and performance, and benefits bone health. Weight-bearing exercise is the most effective type of strength training to maintain strong bones.

Bone growth is stimulated in two ways. The first is the force of a muscle pulling on the bone—muscle contractions against external weights, which happens in strength training. Any exercise that involves your body's weight, free weights, weight machines, or resistance bands creates this type of force by stimulating the development of proteins in muscle cells. Push-ups, modified push-ups, and wall push-ups also are examples.

The second way is ground reaction force—the amount of force exerted against a surface, like a sidewalk, track, or gym floor. Example of exercises that require ground reaction forces are walking, running, and jumping.

Body composition

Our bodies have both lean tissue (muscles, bones, and organs) and fat (essential and nonessential). Body composition—fat mass percentage compared to lean tissue—is important because the percentage of fat mass determines if you are at risk for health problems. A percentage of body fat that is too low could be an indication of malnutrition or under-nutrition. Body fat percentage that is too high increases the risk of cardiovascular disease, diabetes, high blood pressure, and some forms of cancer.

Two measurements that are useful in assessing body fat percentage (but not conclusive) are Body Mass Index (BMI) and waist circumference. BMI is a measure of body fat based on height and weight, but it does not distinguish between lean and fat tissue (see Box 1-6, Body Mass Index). You can calculate your BMI at cdc.gov/healthyweight/assessing/bmi.

Waist circumference indicates where the excessive fat is located—not a mystery for most people—but still does not reveal percentage of body fat. Other measurements, like skin fold, BOD POD (a machine that measures whole body density to determine body composition), and bioelectrical impedance, are more complex, yet more precise. The American College of Sports Medicine provides a guideline for optimal body composition for men and women (see Box 1-7, Body composition: percentage of body fat). Once you know your percentage of body fat, this can tell you how it relates to your overall health.

Research has consistently shown that exercise in general, and strength training in particular, can change body composition in a positive way, although it takes time, effort, and dedication. One of the most recent findings showed that low-intensity resistance

BOX 1-6

Body Mass Index

BODY FAT PERCENTAGE	CATEGORY
< 18.5	underweight
18.5 to 24.9	healthy
25 to 29.9	overweight *
30 to 34.9	grade 1 obesity
35 to 39.9	grade 2 obesity
>40	grade 3 (morbid obesity)

BOX 1-7

Body composition: percentage of body fat		Percentage of body fat					
		AGE: 40-49		AGE: 50-59		AGE: 60+	
PERCENTILE		MEN	WOMEN	MEN	WOMEN	MEN	WOMEN
90	EXCELLENT	13.6	18.5	15.3	21.6	15.3	21.1
80		16.3	21.3	17.9	25.0	18.4	25.1
70	ABOVE AVERAGE	18.1	23.5	19.8	26.2	20.3	27.5
60		19.6	24.9	21.3	28.5	22.0	29.3
50	AVERAGE	21.1	26.4	22.7	30.1	23.5	30.9
40		22.5	28.1	24.1	31.6	25.0	32.5
30	BELOW AVERAGE	24.1	30.1	25.7	33.5	26.7	34.3
20		26.1	32.1	27.5	35.6	28.5	36.6
10	POOR	28.9	35.0	30.3	37.9	31.2	39.3

Resistance training and dietary changes prevent loss of lean body mass

Researchers evaluated the effects of dietary changes and low-intensity resistance exercise training on 41 overweight women, average age of 54. The subjects were assigned to one of three groups for 12 weeks: 1) exercise only, 2) diet only, or 3) exercise combined with dietary changes (fewer calories per day). Those in the diet-only group lost fat in the trunk area of the body. Low-intensity resistance training alone did not affect body composition, but those in the combination exercise/diet group improved muscle strength and prevented further loss of lean body mass.

American Journal of Hypertension, March 2013

training, combined with dietary changes, improved muscle strength and prevented the loss of lean body mass in postmenopausal women (see Box 1-8, "Resistance training and dietary changes prevent loss of lean body mass").

Here is the Centers for Disease Control and Prevention's position on strength training, body composition, and weight management: "The important thing about strength training is the change in body composition. You will gain muscle and most likely decrease body fat, even if your body weight stays the same."

Loss of muscle mass

Age-related loss of muscle mass—called sarcopenia—affects as many as 50 percent of older adults, but noticeable changes can occur earlier in adulthood.

The problems related to sarcopenia, in addition to loss of muscle mass and strength, include issues with mobility, frailty, osteoporosis, falls, and fractures, as well as decreased activity, diabetes, and weight gain. Strength tends to diminish faster than muscle mass, according to a study published in *Frontiers in Physiology.*

The accumulation of physical impairments can eventually result in the loss of physical function and independence. The risk of disability is up to 4.6 times higher in older persons with sarcopenia than in those with normal muscle tissue and strength.

The International Osteoporosis Foundation says that exercise, and in particular resistance training, is extremely effective for preventing sarcopenia, as it affects the neuromuscular system, protein synthesis, and hormones.

After a program of resistance training is introduced, motor neuron firing and protein synthesis (both of which are needed in building muscle mass) increase, even in older adults. These changes suggest that it is possible to rebuild muscle strength, even at an advanced age.

Although some degree of sarcopenia appears to be inevitable with aging, exercise plus dietary changes can reduce the rate of muscle mass and strength loss. A study published in *Osteoporosis International* identified protein and vitamin D as essential factors in muscle health, mass, and function. The report also said that excessive intake of acid-producing foods and acids (red meat, white bread, alcohol, for example), when combined with a low intake of fruits and vegetables, may have a negative effect on muscle and bone health. Finally, it warned that decreases in vitamin B-12 and folic acid intake may impair muscle function.

Diabetes

People with type 2 diabetes have high blood glucose levels that can be lowered by exercise. Exercise increases insulin sensitivity so that cells are better able to use the insulin that is available, according to the American Diabetes Association (ADA).

When muscles contract, a separate mechanism allows cells to take up glucose and use it for energy even in the absence of available insulin.

The ADA and the American College of Sports Medicine issued the following joint statement regarding three types of exercise training as they relate to people who have type 2 diabetes:

◗ **Aerobic exercise training:** "Persons with type 2 diabetes should undertake at least 150 minutes per week of moderate-to-vigorous aerobic exercise spread out across at least three days, with no more than two consecutive days between bouts of aerobic activity."

◗ **Resistance exercise training:** "In addition to aerobic training, persons with type 2 diabetes should undertake moderate-to-vigorous resistance training at least two to three days per week.

◗ **Flexibility training:** Supervised and combined aerobic and resistance training may confer additional health benefits, although milder forms of physical activity, like yoga, have shown mixed results. Persons with type 2 diabetes are encouraged to increase their daily unstructured physical activity. Flexibility training may be included, but should not take the place of other recommended types of physical activity.

A study supporting the inclusion of resistance training in the management of diabetes appeared in the *International Journal of Behavioral Nutrition and Physical Activity* (see Box 1-9, "Resistance training effective in reducing the risk of type 2 diabetes").

The following are summaries of other studies published since the joint ADA and ACSM statement was issued:

◗ Engagement in muscle-strengthening and conditioning activities (resistance exercise, yoga, stretching) is associated with a lower risk of type 2 diabetes in middle-aged and older women. — *PLOS Medicine*, January 14, 2014

◗ Emerging research suggests that resistance training has the power to combat metabolic dysfunction in patients with type 2 diabetes, and seems to be an effective measure to improve overall metabolic health and reduce metabolic risk factors in diabetic patients. —*BioMed Research International*, December 2013

RECENT FINDING BOX 1-9

Resistance training effective in reducing the risk of type 2 diabetes

A team of Australian researchers investigated the effectiveness of multi-component interventions for type 2 diabetes, including diet, aerobic exercise, and resistance training. The study involved more than 1,000 subjects around the world, including the U.S. Diabetes prevention interventions that included aerobic and resistance exercise training, as well as diet, were modestly effective in inducing weight loss and improving factors associated with diabetes, such as impaired fasting glucose and glucose tolerance. The results support the current exercise guidelines for including resistance training in type 2 diabetes prevention.

International Journal of Behavioral Nutrition and Physical Activity, January 15, 2014

Older adults in the best physical condition have the best mental abilities

Researchers at Boston University School of Medicine found that seniors in the best physical condition appear to have the best cognitive abilities, and those with poor physical fitness in their 40s may have lower brain volumes at age 60. Those were two of the findings presented earlier this year, based on data collected from 1,271 participants in the Framingham Offspring Study. The subjects were monitored from the time when their average age was 41 until age 60. Those with a lower fitness level had smaller brain volume, and performed at a lower rate on decision-making function later in life. Every 3.4 units lower exercise capacity, 7.1 mmHg higher exercise diastolic blood pressure, and 8.3 beats per minute higher exercise heart rate in midlife, were approximately equivalent to an additional 0.5 years of brain aging.

Presentation, American Heart Association EPI/Lifestyle Meeting, March 4, 2015

▶ Although exercise is widely recognized as an important component of treatment for type 2 diabetes, emerging research suggests that resistance training may impose powerful and unique benefits. —*Journal of Nutrition and Metabolism*, 2012 Annual Report

▶ Resistance training, similarly to aerobic training, improves metabolic features and insulin sensitivity, and reduces abdominal fat in type 2 diabetic patients. —*Diabetes Care*, April 2012

There are also demonstrated benefits to those with type 1 diabetes, although the evidence is not as conclusive. Type 1 diabetics should consult with their health-care team regarding all aspects of diabetes management, including exercise.

Digestion

Most people are not likely to associate exercise with digestion, but that would be a mistake. Research shows that exercise and digestion are connected in various ways, some of them inside-out (food intake affects energy, performance, strength, and endurance needed to exercise), and others outside-in (exercise affects how the digestive system operates internally). Here are some examples:

▶ Exercise helps the body absorb nutrients more efficiently.

▶ Exercise improves circulation throughout the body, including the digestive tract.

▶ Exercise can help you avoid constipation, bloating, and stomach cramps.

▶ Exercise helps strengthen abdominal muscles, which push digestive waste through the stomach.

▶ Exercise speeds the movement of food through the upper portion of the small intestine, and increases the movements of muscles in the colon.

▶ Exercising on a full stomach can cause digestive distress.

▶ Extremely vigorous exercise (like running for example) and exercise of long duration can have a negative effect on the digestive system.

Mental and emotional health

The evidence supporting exercise as a means of maintaining or improving mental and emotional health is strong (see Box 1-10, "Older adults in the best physical condition have the best mental abilities"), but less compelling when applied to only resistance training. Studies of varying quality have suggested that resistance training is associated with improved memory, cognition, quality of sleep, and self-esteem, and with less depression, chronic fatigue, and anxiety.

It is relatively safe to say that regular exercise in general has a positive effect on both mental and emotional health.

The Centers for Disease Control and Prevention takes this position on the benefits of strength training for emotional health: "Strength training provides similar improvements in depression as antidepressant medications. Currently, it is not known if this is because people feel better when they are stronger, or if strength training produces a helpful biochemical change in the brain. It is most likely a combination of the two. When older adults participate in strength-training programs, their self-confidence and self-esteem improve, which has a strong impact on their overall quality of life."

Weight management/metabolism

While the evidence says resistance training is good for people of all ages, it is not the best type of exercise (alone) for weight loss or weight management. As one exercise scientist said, "It's not that resistance training isn't good for you; it's just not very good at burning fat."

A landmark study conducted at Duke University and published in the *Journal of Applied Physiology* compared aerobic training, resistance training, and a combination of the two in terms of burning fat.

More than 200 overweight or obese adults were assigned to a resistance-training group (three days per week of weight lifting, three sets per day, eight to 12 repetitions per set), aerobic training (12 miles per week), or a combination of weight lifting and aerobic exercise.

Participants in the combination aerobic/resistance training group lost more weight than those who did just resistance training. The resistance-only group actually gained weight, but the gain was attributed to an increase in lean body mass, not fatty tissue.

Aerobic training appeared to be the optimal mode of exercising for reducing fat mass and body mass. A program including resistance training is needed for increasing lean body mass in middle-aged, overweight/obese individuals.

The authors concluded that while no one type of exercise is best for every health benefit, resistance training alone cannot be

BOX 1-11

Do you have trouble with...

	NO ☒	YES ☑
• Opening jars?		
• Getting up from a chair or sofa?		
• Lifting or carrying a bag of groceries or a load of laundry?		
• Opening cellophane food packages?		
• Lifting or holding a baby or young child?		
• Getting luggage out of the trunk of a car?		
• Placing a heavy object on a high shelf?		
• Digging or shoveling in the yard or garden?		
• Starting a gas-powered lawn mower engine?		
• Lifting a bag of mulch or soil?		

RECENT FINDING BOX 1-12

Most effective peer pressure to improve fitness may come from spouse

Research showed that if one spouse improves his or her exercise program, the other spouse is significantly more likely to follow suit. Data on more than 15,000 middle-aged adults in four states revealed that when a wife met recommended levels of exercise after a visit with her doctor, her husband was 70 percent more likely to meet those levels at subsequent visits than the husbands of women who were physically less active. When a husband met recommended levels, his wife was 40 percent more likely to meet the levels at follow-up visits. The researchers concluded that the best peer pressure regarding an exercise program might come from a spouse.

Presentation, American Heart Association EPI/Lifestyle Meeting, March 4. 2015

expected to make a significant difference in decreased fat mass or body weight.

Functional fitness

As important as resistance training is for all of the health issues just described, the most practical benefits involve activities of daily living. "Functional fitness," or "functional strength," is the term used to describe strength that helps us perform the activities we do every day in a manner that is efficient, painless (for the most part), and reduces the risk of injury.

It almost always involves more than one muscle or muscle group. Traditional strength training tends to isolate muscle groups, but muscles of the upper arms made stronger don't necessarily help you perform a task that requires strength in the arms, shoulders, and core (for example, bending to pick up an object).

Box 1-11, "Do you have trouble with..." offers 10 examples of daily activities that require functional strength. Check the items that apply. If you answer "yes" to one or more of the questions, you may have lost strength and might benefit from strength training, functional fitness training, or both.

Demands of a resistance training program

If "sticking with it" is the number one challenge of a successful resistance training program, challenge number 1-A might be making a commitment to begin one. For some, motivation to begin and adhere to a program might be the same.

There is no all-purpose motivational tool. Some people—like those rare individuals who abruptly stop smoking, or make a dramatic change in their diet to lose weight—just do it, probably for reasons that would not necessarily motivate others. Still, others are motivated by health or potential health concerns, self-esteem, the challenge, approval of others, or peer pressure.

Two studies provide documentation of what has worked. One with a surprising result involved peer pressure. The other addressed motivational factors that prompted successful exercisers to begin and stay with their programs.

At Johns Hopkins University, data presented in March 2015 on more than 15,000 people showed that the most effective peer pressure for changing exercise habits may come "from the person sitting across the table from you at breakfast—your spouse."

Husbands were 70 percent more likely to reach recommended

fitness levels after their wives had been advised by a doctor to engage in a more demanding exercise program. Wives were 40 percent more likely to follow their husbands' leads in picking up the pace (see Box 1-12, "Most effective peer pressure to improve fitness may come from spouse").

A study conducted in Canada and published in 2014 explored factors that influence adherence to regular exercise in middle-aged women (see Box 1-13, "Daily routines, positive feelings make adherence to exercise more likely"). The most common factors that enabled success were 1) daily routines that accommodated exercise; 2) anticipating positive feelings associated with exercise (as one researcher put it, "seeing exercise as an 'I get to' activity rather than an 'I have to' activity"); and 3) being accountable to someone else, like a friend, an instructor, a group, or a spouse.

Cost

Cost may not be the most important factor in deciding to begin a program, but it is understandably a consideration. The cost of an exercise program can come in three forms: 1) apparel; 2) equipment, if you choose to conduct your program at home; and 3) supervised instruction (see Chapter 2 for detailed information.)

The best-case scenario for a do-it-yourself program is low cost—perhaps $15 or less for a box of resistance bands. Worst-case scenario is hundreds or even thousands of dollars, spread over months and years for people who invest in high-end strength-training machines they don't use, membership to gyms they don't visit, and/or personal trainers they do not utilize.

Time

Time commitment comes in three levels. At the first level is a single resistance training session, which can easily be completed in an hour (and in some cases, only 30 minutes). The exact length depends on the number of exercises per session, the number of repetitions, the number of sets, and the time between exercises. (Guidelines for each are given in Chapters 2, 3, and 4.)

The second-level time commitment is the number of sessions per week. That one is easy. Most of the major health and fitness-related organizations, including the Centers for Disease Control and Prevention, the National Health Institutes, and the American

RECENT FINDING   BOX 1-13

Daily routines, positive feelings make adherence to exercise more likely

Canadian researchers identified six broad themes and three sub-themes that influenced women between the ages of 40 and 62 to adhere to regular exercise: 1) a daily structure that incorporated physical activity, 2) anticipation of positive feelings associated with exercise, also called intrinsic motivation, and 3) accountability to an individual or group of people. Unlike other studies, lack of time, environmental challenges (bad weather), and menopausal symptoms were not identified as barriers to exercise. The most significant barriers were other demands, like disrupted daily structure, and self-sacrifice (the feeling that other life factors were more important than benefits to be gained from exercise).

BMC Women's Health, March 26, 2014

BOX 1-14

ACSM guidelines for resistance exercise

- Adults should train each major muscle group two or three days each week, using a variety of exercises and equipment.

- Very light or light intensity is best for older people or previously sedentary adults starting exercise.

- Two to four sets of each exercise will help adults improve strength and power.

- For each exercise, 8-12 repetitions improve strength and power, 10-15 repetitions improve strength in middle-aged and older people starting exercise, and 15-20 repetitions improve muscular endurance.

- Adults should wait at least 48 hour between resistance training sessions.

College of Sports Medicine, recommend two to four resistance-training sessions per week on non-consecutive days.

The third-level commitment is long term and often the most difficult, as one-half of people who begin exercise programs drop out within six months (*Clinical Interventions in Aging*, February 14, 2014). But there is good news: If you can make it past six months, you have a good chance to be a regular (resistance training) exerciser for life.

Missing a session here and there is not a problem, but missing regular sessions is since strength gains can be lost quickly among older adults. Schedule your sessions and do your best to follow it, instead of only exercising "when you have time."

Effort

Resistance training is work. It can be fun and rewarding, but gaining strength requires effort beyond normal daily activities. It's okay to get hot, sweaty, tired, and possibly sore after the first few workouts. The concept of progressive resistance implies that you keep challenging muscles and muscle groups to get stronger by exerting muscle force against resistance. From an exercise science perspective, resistance training is about overload, progression, and specificity.

Overload is the stress placed on your body when physical activity is greater than usual. The body adapts to muscle- and bone-strengthening activities by making the bones and muscles stronger to meet the new challenges.

Progression refers to small, progressive changes in overload that help the body adapt to additional stress, while minimizing the risk of injury.

Specificity means the benefits of strength training are specific to the areas of the body doing the work. For example, running is not going to increase upper body strength. Instead, you need resistance training exercises like arm curls, shoulder shrugs, and push-ups.

After working out, the body begins to repair and replace damaged fibers, forming new muscle protein strands (myofibrils) that result in stronger and sometimes bigger muscle tissue (although not that much bigger in females because they don't have the same level of testosterone as men). Muscle rebuilding takes time—48 hours between moderate and heavy lifting sessions.

Begin your program with a weight or other resistance you can lift, push, pull, or move for eight to 12 repetitions while using proper form. (A repetition is the number of times you perform a single exercise movement—like a curl or shrug.) Complete one set of eight to 12 reps before resting.

When you have achieved that goal, add another set, then consider adding a third set later. There is no evidence that going beyond two to four sets (unless you are also trying to improve power) provides added benefits. More is not always better. It won't make you stronger and may increase the risk of injury. Box 1-14, "ACSM guidelines for resistance exercise," outlines the ACSM's exact guidelines for strength training.

Results will happen, but take time. For instance, Tufts University research showed that a 60-year-old adult who resistance trains can gain two or three pounds of muscle in six months to a year. Absolute strength gains can be observed sooner, but changes still require a certain time span.

Strength plus power

Power training is not usually at the top of the to-do list for older adults. Most people familiar with weight training, a type of strength training that uses only free weights for resistance, associate "power" with common movements like "power lifts," "power cleans," or "power jerks." In other words, power lifting movements. The average person might also associate power training with younger adults using heavy barbells, often to prepare for athletic performance or Olympic weight lifting.

But power training should be a larger part of strength training. Various studies have shown an association between power and quality of life, like hitting the brakes quicker in a car, as well as gains in strength, performing daily tasks, fall prevention, and increased walking speed (see Box 1-15, "Increasing the velocity of power training could make older adults safer").

If strength is the ability to exert force against resistance, power is the same concept, but with speed. It's one thing to have enough lower body strength to walk leisurely across a street when signal says, "Walk." It's quite another to make it across that street when the caution light blinks and cars approach. A person in that situation needs both strength and power.

A review of studies published in the *International Journal of Exercise Science* concluded that strength and power training in older adults can both "significantly improve functional

RECENT FINDING BOX 1-15

Increasing the velocity of power training could make older adults safer

Two University of Missouri researchers compared changes in peak power as a result of high-speed power training in older adults versus traditional slow-speed strength training. Eighty-four adults whose ages ranged from 68 to 71 were randomly assigned to a high-speed group, a slow-speed group, or a control group for a period of 12 weeks. Improvement in muscle power and strength occurred in both intervention groups, but the group that experimented with resistance training at higher speeds produced significantly greater changes. The authors concluded that high-speed power training should be implemented with older adults to improve speed of movement needed for functional tasks related to safety, such as crossing a busy intersection, and fall prevention.

Journal of Strength & Conditioning Research, March 2014

Combined endurance and strength training improves muscle quality in older adults

Researchers at the Mayo Clinic College of Medicine and their colleagues at other institutions found that combining endurance training with resistance training resulted in muscle strength and quality improvements, regardless of age. Sixty-five adults between the ages of 18 and 65 were randomly assigned to one of three training interventions—cycling (for aerobic endurance), resistance training (four sets, eight to 10 repetitions), or combined aerobic and resistance training over an eight-week period. Body composition, muscle strength, and peak oxygen uptake, as well as muscle biopsies, were used to measure changes before and after the trials. All three interventions improved body composition, cardiorespiratory fitness, and muscle strength, and most training-induced improvements were independent of age. The combined program resulted in the strongest improvements in muscle quality and strength in older subjects, which could be a significant finding for the treatment of sarcopenia (loss of muscle mass associated with aging).

Journal of Clinical & Endocrinological Metabolism, February 2015

BOX 1-17

Days per week required for total fitness

FITNESS COMPONENT	DAYS PER WEEK
Resistance/Strength	2-3, non-consecutive days
Flexibility	At least 2-3 days
Aerobic	5 days (moderate intensity) 3 days (vigorous intensity)
Balance	2-3 days

performance," and suggested that power training may be more effective than strength training in that regard.

However, incorporating power training into the early stages of strength training, which is usually done with slow, controlled movement, could be troublesome. The last thing a middle-aged-plus adult (unaccustomed to exercising) should do is move somewhat heavy weights at a fast speed. It's the perfect recipe for an injury.

The solution is to gradually introduce power training into a strength-training routine, using movements that mimic those of daily activities. One example of an exercise that incorporates several fitness components—lower body strength, core strength, power, flexibility, and balance—is getting out of a chair.

The simple act of going from a sitting to standing position is slow and difficult for those who might have a strength deficit. Performing sit-to-stand-sit repetitions at a slow speed would build strength. Doing the same exercise at a faster pace would build strength and power.

Strength plus muscle endurance

There is a difference between muscle strength, muscle power, and muscle endurance. Strength is the ability to exert force against resistance, or in simpler terms, how much work your muscles can do at one time. Power refers to the speed or explosiveness of muscle movement—strength plus speed in short bursts. Muscle endurance is how long you can use your muscles during one training session or episode.

To gain only strength, you would begin exercising (lifting, for example) at lower resistance and gradually increase the load. To gain power, you would increase the speed at which you move weights. To improve muscle endurance, you would use lower-resistance weights, but increase the number of repetitions dramatically (see Box 1-16, "Combined endurance and strength training improves muscle quality in older adults").

Putting it all together

A recurring theme in the Stay Fit Series is the importance of incorporating exercises and activities to improve all four fitness components—strength, balance, aerobic fitness, and flexibility. There are enough days in a week and enough combinations of exercises to work on each area, some on the same day. Box 1-17, "Days per week required for total fitness," shows each fitness component and the minimum number of days per week needed to maintain your fitness status or improve it.

By combining programs on the same day, you can, for example, do 30-plus minutes of aerobic training, followed by 30-plus minutes of resistance training. The order doesn't matter, according to a study published in the April 2014 issue of the *European Journal of Applied Physiology* (Box 1-18, "Order of strength and aerobic training has no effect on performance or recovery"). It's more a matter of preference than exercise science.

Flexibility exercises can be included during warm ups and cool downs for aerobic training. Balance exercises require just a few minutes of time, and can be done almost every day at home, regardless of what else is on your schedule.

What's next?

There are a few details to take care of before you begin your program. Chapter 2, *Before You Begin*, will help you work through this pre-exercise to-do-checklist.

RECENT FINDING   BOX 1-18

Order of strength and aerobic training has no effect on performance or recovery

A European research group tested 12 men to determine if the order of exercise—aerobic first, then strength training, or strength training first, then aerobic—had an effect on performance or recovery. To test endurance (aerobic fitness), the men performed steady-state cycling. For strength, the exercise was leg presses. The training was conducted over a 24-week period. No significant differences in strength development or recovery were observed, regardless of the order in which the exercise was performed on the same days.

European Journal of Applied Physiology, April 2014

❷ BEFORE YOU BEGIN

Before beginning any new fitness program, including resistance training, check with your doctor. Explain what the program will involve in terms of exercise type, intensity, instruction, and supervision. You will likely get one of these three responses, although not with these exact words:

1. Great. It'll be good for you.
2. Go with the program, but with certain restrictions.
3. A strength- or power-training program is not advisable at this time, but may be appropriate at a later date (probably after you have fully recovered from your injury, surgical procedure, or illness).

Limitations

Many conditions could present risks or exercise limitations, but in almost every case, a resistance-training program can be modified to fit individual needs. The following are examples, but they do not necessarily or automatically disqualify you from modified strength-training exercises. Again, check with your doctor. Chapter 3 includes 14 ways to modify exercises (see page 42).

- Blood clots
- Cardiovascular disease family history
- Chest pain
- Chronic lung disease
- Diabetes
- Eye injuries/surgery
- Foot/ankle sores
- Heart disease
- Heart palpitations
- Hernia
- Hypertension
- Infections
- Knee/hip arthritis
- Pain walking after a fall
- Recent or chronic orthopedic injuries
- Shortness of breath
- Smoking

How do you compare?

The following informal self tests can be done at home and give you a rough idea of your current strength or lack of strength, power, and other fitness components. They can also double as strength-training exercises. They are safe, but you need to be careful. It's okay to practice each move before taking the tests.

30-second chair stand

● Measures: Lower body strength, core strength, and muscle endurance.

● Equipment: Sturdy, straight-back chair with no arms, stopwatch.

● Instructions:

- Sit in the chair with your arms crossed at the wrists.
- When your test partner says "Go" complete as many sit-stand repetitions as you can in 30 seconds.
- Don't use your hands to push off. Rise to a full stand then sit all the way down (no touch and rise).
- Box 2-1, "Normal range scores: 30-second chair stand," gives normal range scores for men and women 60 years and older.

BOX 2-1

Normal range scores: 30-second chair stand

AGE	MEN	WOMEN
60-64	14-19	12-17
65-69	12-18	11-16
70-74	12-17	10-15
75-79	11-17	10-15
80-84	10-15	9-14
85-89	8-14	8-13
90-94	7-12	4-11

Arm curl

● Measures: Upper body strength.

● Equipment: An eight-pound weight for men; a five-pound weight for women (to conform to established testing norms), straight-back chair with no arms, stopwatch.

● Instructions:

- Begin in a sitting position, arm straight down holding the dumbbell.
- When your test partner says "Go" complete as many curls as you can in 30 seconds.
- Move in a controlled manner, and touch the upper arm with the hand holding the weight with each repetition.
- Box 2-2, "Normal range scores: Arm curl," gives normal range scores for men and women 60 years and older.

BOX 2-2

Normal range scores: Arm curl

AGE	MEN	WOMEN
60-64	16-22	13-19
65-69	15-21	12-18
70-74	14-21	12-17
75-79	13-19	11-17
80-84	13-19	10-16
85-89	11-17	10-15
90-94	10-14	8-13

Timed up-and-go

● Measures: Combination of strength (getting up), power (moving with speed), balance, and agility.

● Equipment: Chair, cone/marker eight feet from chair, stopwatch.

● Instructions:

- Begin in a sitting position, hands on thighs, feet flat on floor, one foot slightly forward.
- When your test partner says "Go" and starts the stopwatch, rise and walk as quickly as possible around the marker and back to your seat.
- When you are seated, your test partner stops the watch and records your time to the nearest tenth of a second.
- Box 2-3, "Normal range scores: Timed up-and-go," gives normal range scores for men and women 60 years and older.

BOX 2-3

Normal range scores: Timed up-and-go

AGE	MEN	WOMEN
60-64	5.6-3.8	6.0-4.4
65-69	5.7-4.3	6.4-4.8
70-74	6.0-4.2	7.1-4.9
75-79	7.2-4.6	7.4-5.2
80-84	7.6-5.2	8.7-5.7
85-89	8.9-5.3	9.6-6.2
90-94	10.0-6.2	11.5-7.3

Finding a program

Anyone can begin a strength-training program at home. All you need is the right equipment, a little space, and an exercise guide (like this Special Report) or program to follow.

Although not a requirement, having a workout partner is a good idea for most people beginning a strength-training program. A friend, spouse, or other family member can assist with some exercises and share the same equipment. A workout partner also helps relieve the monotony of doing repetitive exercises.

Community centers and wellness facilities offer strength-training programs where others work out, but each person has to do most of the work alone. The National Council on Aging (www.ncoa.org) endorses programs that are proven to produce measurable health benefits, including strength training for older adults. The programs are administered through providers in local communities. They include:

▶ Active Living Every Day (ALED) uses a ALED book, and offers online support for participants.

▶ EnhanceFitness involves one-hour group classes that include stretching, flexibility, balance, low-impact aerobics, and strength training.

▶ EnhanceWellness is a self-care wellness program that involves a nurse and social worker who help develop an individual health and fitness plan.

▶ Fit and Strong combines flexibility, strength training, and aerobic walking with health education for older adults with lower extremity osteoarthritis.

▶ Healthy Moves for Aging Well is an in-home physical activity intervention for sedentary seniors.

▶ Walk with Ease is an Arthritis Foundation program that helps participants meet their needs, stay motivated, manage pain, and exercise safely.

▶ S.A.I.L. (Stay Active and Independent for Life), offered by UCLA, is an evidence-based flexibility, balance, strengthening, and aerobic exercise and education program, focused on fall prevention in the senior population.

Other facilities

Colleges and universities, wellness centers, YMCAs, hospitals, and physical therapy clinics also offer fitness and strength-training programs. Here, a fitness specialist conducts an assessment, recommends a program, instructs you on resistance training technique, and keeps an eye on you (and others) while you exercise.

Expect a one-time assessment cost of $50 to $100, then a monthly fee of $7 to $10 per session or $40 to $80 per month that should include two to three sessions per week (prices vary with location). Some programs are offered free to older adults or may be covered by health insurance (check with your provider).

Personal trainers

At home or in a fitness facility, personal trainers are another option for some. They can design and supervise individual strength-training programs, and you will be charged by the hour, or by a flat fee for a specified number of sessions. A National Strength and Conditioning Association survey found this costs an average of $50 per hour, but prices vary widely.

The advantages of having a personal trainer are expertise, instruction, efficiency, accountability, supervision, and motivation. The disadvantages are cost and difficulty in finding a trainer who is qualified and with whom you are comfortable.

The rate of turnover among personal trainers is high. Try to find one who is a career personal trainer instead of a person who does it part time or who is transitioning from one position to another. Get references and ask friends or family members for recommendations.

Make sure personal trainers are certified by one of the nationally recognized agencies—the National Academy of Sports Medicine, American College of Sports Medicine, National Strength and Conditioning Association, or American Council on Exercise.

Types of equipment

The most available and least expensive type of resistance-training equipment is you. Body-weight exercises can help any muscle or muscle group become stronger. Entire strength-training programs can be designed using only body-weight exercises.

Push-ups, sit-ups, and pull-ups are examples of the classic, old school body-weight exercises, but several varieties of the "Superman" exercise (see Box 2-4, "Superman") are now used to strengthen core muscles.

SUPERMAN   BOX 2-4

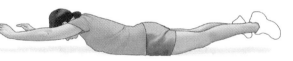

"Superman" is a floor exercise that uses your body weight to strengthen the core muscles from the shoulders to the hips.

STABILITY BALL ARM/KNEE LIFT

BOX 2-5

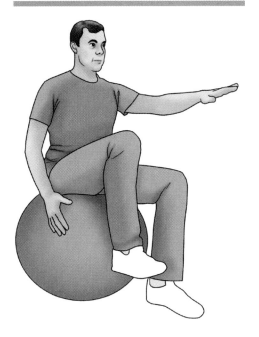

Stability balls force the person to use core muscles, even if they are exercising other muscle groups.

Free weights

A free weight is one that is not attached to an apparatus. Dumbbells (handweights) and barbells are the two most frequently used free weights, but dumbbells (not barbells) are a good match for beginning strength-trainers and older adults. Begin with two- to three-pound weights for each hand, and gradually move up to dumbbells that weigh five pounds or more.

Vinyl-covered dumbbells are often easier to grip and hold than traditional metal dumbbells. They cost from $80 to $125 for a complete set. You can get started with light-weight dumbbells, if desired, for much less. Entry-level exercisers need a set that includes weights of one to eight pounds (with increments in between).

Kettlebells have become an increasingly popular free weight. They are cast iron weights of between five and 100-plus pounds, and used for a variety of swinging and pulling motions that involve momentum and centrifugal force. If you are a middle-aged or older adult and want to exercise with a free weight, stick with the dumbbells for now and consider kettlebells later.

Another equipment option is home-made free weights, such as water-filled milk cartons, or vegetable cans that weigh between one and three pounds. Any household object can substitute for a dumbbell, but for safety's safe, make sure it's something with a handle.

CHOOSING THE RIGHT SIZE STABILITY BALL

BOX 2-6

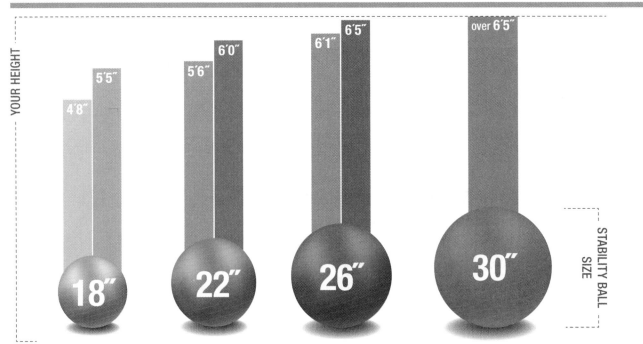

Stability balls

Stability balls are excellent for stretching and strengthening core-related muscles, but they can be used with weights for other muscle groups, as well (see Box 2-5, "Stability Ball Arm/ Knee Lift"). The instability of sitting or lying on the ball forces one to use his or her core muscles to keep the body level.

It's important to use a stability ball that is the right size. When sitting on one, your thighs should be parallel to the floor. Box 2-6 "Choosing the right size stability ball," shows how to match individual height with the size of the ball. Prices begin at about $15.

The greater the inflation of the ball, the less stable it is as a base, so the more effort from core muscles are needed to stabilize it. Less air is better for beginners and intermediates.

Resistance bands

Resistance bands are inexpensive, space-saving, stretchable bands or tubes made from natural or synthetic rubber. Use them almost anywhere to work through a range of movements against resistance. Curls, shrugs, leg swings, and squats are examples (see Box 2-7, "Resistance band squats").

However, there are limitations. Bands get old and lose their resistance feature, the amount of resistance is hard to measure (with free weights, you know exactly how much you are lifting), and the amount of resistance changes throughout the exercise motion.

Colors indicating amount of resistance vary among manufacturers, but with all of them the force is directly related to the percentage of elongation. The amount of resistance ranges from 3.3 pounds to about 22 pounds.

Check the bands before every workout for nicks and tears, don't wear rings while using them, and avoid storing them in extremely hot or cold temperatures. Replace them every three to four months. Resistance bands are inexpensive—about $10 for a box of basic bands to $100 for bands with added features like handles (see Box 2-8, "Resistance bands with handles").

Medicine balls

Medicine balls can help develop strength, power, and balance, but they are most effective for dynamic movement (strength plus speed of movement). Traditional medicine ball exercises were designed primarily for core muscles, but now they are

RESISTANCE BAND SQUATS · BOX 2-7

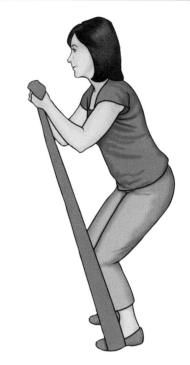

Resistance bands can be used for upper and lower body strength training.

RESISTANCE BANDS WITH HANDLES · BOX 2-8

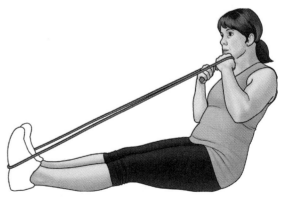

Resistance bands with handles cost more, but may be worth the price as they are easier to grip..

Chair-based exercises enhance strength and flexibility in older adults

In Great Britain, a review study of professional literature was undertaken to address the purpose and benefits of chair-based exercises (CBE). The researchers found that CBE is an appropriate form of resistance and flexibility training for older and frail adults. Among the findings, 1) using a chair during exercise promotes stability in both sitting and standing positions; 2) CBE should be used as a starting point to begin a more challenging program; 3) CBE should be a component in which a progression of exercise is encouraged, and 4) CBE should be used to respond to the changing needs of older adults.

BMC Geriatrics, May 19, 2014

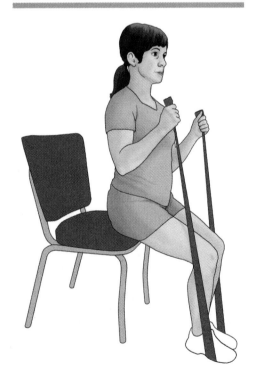

Resistance bands can be incorporated into chair-based exercises.

also used for other muscle groups and can be incorporated into strength-training programs. Weights range from two to 30 pounds, and having several balls of varying weights allows for a variety of exercises and differences in exercise load. Prices begin at about $20.

Cuff weights

Cuff weights with Velcro-type straps wrap around wrists and ankles to provide resistance during movement. Some have a single weight, but most allow to you to add and remove small weight plates (one pound each) to increase or decrease the load. They are particularly effective for people who might have trouble gripping a dumbbell or similar weight, but who would benefit from performing upper body exercises with weights attached to their wrists or ankles. A single cuff weight costs less than $15; a complete set is $100 or more.

Chairs (for chair-based exercises)

If you need extra support or lack mobility, chair-based exercises might be a way to perform strength-training exercises. The concept was confirmed by a study published in *BMC Geriatrics* (see Box 2-9, "Chair-based exercises enhance strength and flexibility in older adults"). From a sitting position, examples include leg extensions and arm curls. Box 2-10, "Resistance band seated curls," illustrates a method of incorporating resistance bands into a chair-based routine. Any kind of chair will work as long as it's sturdy, not too light, and has a straight back for support.

Weight machines

Weight machines are for people working out at wellness or fitness centers, and for more experienced exercisers. They are not for people beginning a strength-training program at home. Wait until you are more certain of your commitment and strength training goals before investing in weight machines.

The advantages include focusing on one muscle group at a time, performing an exercise through a specific range of motion, controlling movement, and using proper form throughout the lift.

The disadvantages are the cost (a few hundred to thousands of dollars), the lack of "functional fitness" movements, the emphasis on one muscle group instead of simultaneous muscle group movements (which can lead to muscle imbalance), and difficulty in adding small amounts of weight (most machines can be adjusted, but in increments of five to 10 pounds at a time).

Complementary forms of exercise

Yoga, tai chi, and Pilates are forms of exercise defined by the National Center for Complementary and Alternative Medicine (NCCAM) as alternative or complementary. All three have gained immense popularity in the United States in the past two decades.

The National Center for Health Statistics reports that more than 21 million Americans, including three percent of those aged 65 and older, have participated in yoga in the past year (see Box 2-11, "Twenty-one million Americans have done yoga during the past year"). More than two million people in the country engage in tai chi, and as many as eight million sign up for Pilates classes annually.

All three forms of exercise provide health and fitness benefits, but their contributions to strength and power depend on the type of yoga, tai chi, or Pilates exercises, movements, and poses performed. Their direct associations with strength development are difficult to measure, but not impossible.

A study in the *Journal of Aging and Physical Activity* found that yoga resulted in moderate improvements in gait, balance, flexibility, weight loss, and lower body strength. The *International Journal of Yoga* reported that yoga enhances muscular strength and flexibility.

As with traditional forms of strength training, improvement though yoga, tai chi, and Pilates comes only when they involve the principles of overload, progression, and specificity. None of the three basic forms incorporate movements that would increase power.

Yoga

Yoga is not a single exercise program, but rather a mind/body series of movements, postures, breathing techniques, and meditation/relaxation. There are more than 20 styles, including Hatha yoga, which is the form most often used in the United States and Europe. Other popular styles include Iyengar, Ashtanga, Kundalini, and Bikram. Here is a more detailed look at each.

Twenty-one million Americans have done yoga during the past year

Two new government surveys revealed that yoga is becoming increasingly popular among adults in the U.S. More than 10 percent of adults say they have tried yoga, tai chi, or qi gong, but yoga accounts for most of the increase. Although only one percent of older adults had tried the mind-body activity 10 years ago, three percent now have had the experience. Overall, 21 million Americans have tried yoga in the past year. The survey results identified trends only, not reasons why certain alternative or complementary practices are more popular than others.

National Health Statistics Reports, February 10, 2015

BOX 2-12

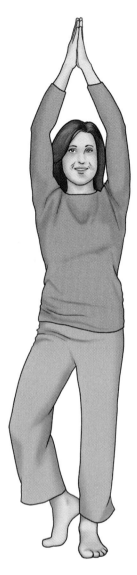

Hatha yoga focuses on basic poses, like Tree Pose, to improve balance and flexibility, and relieve stress.

▶ **Hatha** itself incorporates simple poses (see Box 2-12, "Yoga"), called asanas, that flow from one to the next. Participants are allowed to move at their own pace. One of the main benefits is controlled breathing, or improving oxygenation of the body to alleviate stress.

▶ **Iyengar** is characterized by attention to detail in poses, poses held for longer periods of time, and using props, such as chairs, straps, belts, blankets, blocks, and pillows, to compensate for a lack of flexibility. Iyengar yoga has been called meditation in action. Its benefits are said to include muscle toning, tension elimination, and easing chronic pain, as well as to "strengthen weak areas and stretch tight ones."

▶ **Ashtanga**, also called power yoga, is popular among athletes because of its emphasis on developing strength, flexibility, and stamina. The sequence of poses range from simple to difficult, and students move quickly from one pose to another. Poses include combinations of standing, sitting, back extensions, inversions, balancing, and twisting. Ashtanga does not reply on props for support and is often not advised for beginners and those with flexibility issues.

▶ **Kundalini** is a gentler form of yoga that focuses on mind, body, and emotion, and incorporates poses, body locks, chanting, meditation, visualization, and guided relaxation to achieve its goals.

▶ **Bikram** (also known as "hot yoga") is a 90-minute program performed in heated environments (100-plus degrees Fahrenheit), where 26 poses are performed in a specific order. The exercises are described as physical and intense, designed to raise the heart rate and exercise muscles to a point of fatigue. They are recommended only for extremely fit individuals, and should be avoided by most older adults and all beginning exercisers.

The NCCAM provides the following guidelines for those considering yoga as a form of exercise:

- Do not use yoga to replace conventional medical care.
- Talk to your doctor before beginning a program, especially if you have a medical condition.
- Ask a trusted healthcare provider to recommend a yoga instructor.
- Choose a yoga style that best fits your ability.
- Advise all of your healthcare providers about complementary practices you use, including yoga.

Tai chi

Tai chi is a combination of relaxation, meditation, deep breathing and slow, continuous exercises called forms. The number of forms ranges from 18 to more than 100. Newcomers can begin with one brief (five-minute) session and gradually increase the number and duration of sessions each week.

Tai chi can improve balance, lower the risk of falls, and provide a sense of well-being. Reputable health institutions associate tai chi with less joint pain and better aerobic capacity, energy, stamina, and flexibility, but conclusive evidence regarding tai chi and strength is hard to find.

An often cited study was conducted at Stanford University and published in *Alternative Therapies in Health and Medicine*. Here, 39 women, average age 66, with below-average fitness and at least one cardiovascular risk factor, took 36 tai chi classes over the course of 12 weeks. Tests taken before and after the trial showed that the subjects significantly increased strength and flexibility in the upper and lower body.

Tai chi is safe for most people and effective for specific goals (balance, fall prevention, feeling of well-being). While its value for strength training is still debatable, it is not a way to improve power. People with the following conditions should consult a physician before enrolling in a tai chi program:

- osteoporosis
- chest pain with minimal exertion
- severe shortness of breath
- dizziness or fainting spells
- uncontrolled high blood pressure
- gait and balance disorders

Pilates

Pilates is generally recognized as a means of building strength in core muscles, which has a direct or indirect effect on other muscle groups and is particularly beneficial for improving posture. It consists of 25 to 50 low-impact strength, flexibility, and endurance movements, most of which are performed on the floor, a mat, or specially designed Pilates equipment called reformers. Programs can be individualized for beginners and older adults.

A study in the *Journal of Strength & Conditioning Research* suggested that individuals can improve their muscular endurance and flexibility using relatively low-intensity Pilates exercises that do not require equipment or a high degree of skill. Other studies have shown that Pilates may be useful in regaining strength following debilitating conditions.

Even so, support in the scientific and medical communities for Pilates appears to be hindered, not necessarily because of the practice itself, but by a lack of clinical studies.

As with yoga and tai chi, talk with your doctor before beginning a Pilates program. It is not recommended or should be modified for people who have high blood pressure, a risk of blood clots, severe osteoporosis, or a herniated disc.

Apparel

Workout clothes vary with the activity. For traditional resistance training, all you need are comfortable shorts, tops, and sneakers. For some exercises—yoga and Pilates, for example—most people prefer tight-fitting, stretchable pants (and/or tops) that don't bunch up or slip on mats. Comfort is important in lifting weights or using weight machines, so loose-fitting tops and bottoms are okay as long as they don't interfere with the exercise or get caught in machines.

Proper footwear is important, but high cost does not necessarily mean better quality. Basic sneakers and training shoes are available in the $50 to $100 range. More important considerations are fit, traction (to avoid slipping), lateral support, comfort, durability, and a design that complements your resistance exercise of choice.

Fashionable colors and styles elevate the price, but don't necessarily enhance the experience. However, never buy shoes off the rack. Make sure to get professionally fitted at a running or other specialty store to ensure you buy shoes that fit your arch and foot width. Also, most athletic shoes should be purchased a half-size larger than your regular, everyday footwear.

Studio wraps for yoga and Pilates are less expensive than shoes, and no-slip socks are a consideration, but talk with friends or the instructor before investing a lot of money in footwear. You can always upgrade later.

Weight gloves for resistance training are available, but unless you need padded gloves to protect your hands, they are not must-have accessories.

Compression sleeves for arms and calves are designed to increase circulation in an area of the body. Better blood flow decreases the likelihood of swelling, but unless you are already using them for medical reasons, there is probably no reason to use them during resistance training. Ask your doctor.

Nutrition and strength

As mentioned in Chapter 1, age-related loss of muscle mass and muscle strength is a particular concern among middle-aged and older adults. Maintaining and building muscle and bone strength requires a combination of strength training plus three specific nutritional factors—protein, vitamin D, and intake of fruits and vegetables.

Protein

Protein is a building block for muscle and bone health and helps support the growth and recovery of body tissue after exercise. Current United States Department of Agriculture (USDA) dietary guidelines for Americans suggest men age 50 to 70 consume 56 grams (g) of protein per day, while women should eat 46 g. (Men and women have the same protein requirements per kilogram of body weight, but men usually weigh more than women, so they require more protein.)

Of course, these are estimates, and an individual's requirements depend on factors like height, weight, past medical history, and activity level.

To find your individual protein number, convert your weight to kilograms (kg) by dividing that number by 2.2 and then multiplying that figure by 0.8. For instance a 150-pound person would weight 68 kg and thus need a minimum of 54.4 g of protein per day. You should increase this amount by about 1.2 to 1.5 grams when you exercise.

While lean meats like beef, chicken, and fish are popular protein sources, you can also opt for plant sources like beans, legumes, nuts, seeds, quinoa, soy, and leafy greens (like broccoli), which offer more dietary variety. A scoop of whey or vegan protein powder added to a smoothie or mixed into oatmeal or yogurt also can help supplement your intake.

Vitamin D

Vitamin D helps fuel muscle growth and is necessary for calcium absorption in order to keep bones strong and healthy. Adequate vitamin D comes with safe exposure to sunlight and/or food or supplementation, if required. Sensible sun exposure is 10 to 20 minutes on the arms, legs, and face (or approximately 50 percent of your body), two or three times a week. Vitamin D is naturally present in few foods. Cod liver oil is a rich source, as is some oily fish, such as tuna and salmon. Most milk, orange juice, yogurt, cheese, cereals, breads, and soy drinks are fortified with vitamin D. Check with your doctor before taking any vitamin D supplement. The recommended dietary allowances for vitamin D are:

- 600 international units (IU) for men and women age 51 to 70
- 800 IU for those older than age 70
- 800 to 1000 IU for those who are vitamin D deficient

A blood test from your doctor can determine if you are deficient. It is best to get tested in the winter or early spring when vitamin D levels are often the lowest due to reduced sunlight exposure.

Fruits and vegetables

Excessive intake of acid-producing foods, when combined with a low intake of fruits and vegetables, may have a negative effect on muscle and bone health.

The USDA recommends two cups of fruits per day for people 51 years and older who get less than 30 minutes of moderate physical activity per day beyond normal activities. Those who are more active may be able to consume more while staying within calorie needs.

The USDA recommends two-and-a-half cups of vegetables per day for men 51, and older and two cups for women. Again, those who are more active can consume more.

Same-day eating and exercise

Three organizations—the American College of Sports Medicine, the Mayo Clinic, and the American Heart Association—give the following suggestions regarding same-day nutrition and exercise in general. While these are not for strength training specifically, they can be used as a guideline for all strength-training workouts.

Before

Eat at least an hour before mild-to-moderate exercise with the emphasis on carbohydrates, and include foods such as whole-grain cereals, bread, juices, water, coffee with breakfast, fat-free yogurt, pancakes, waffles, and fruits.

Eat large meals at least three to four hours before vigorous exercise, small meals (more than a snack) at least two to three hours before you begin, and snacks (apples, bananas) an hour prior to exercise.

After

After strenuous exercise, the American Heart Association recommends refueling with fluids (water or water blended with 100 percent fruit juice, carbohydrates (the main fuel for muscles), and protein (to repair and grow muscle tissue.)

Among the suggested foods are whole-grain English muffins, bagels, crackers, low-fat chocolate milk, juice-water blend, energy bars, low-fat granola bars, yogurt, fruits, smoothies, vegetables, peanut butter sandwiches, pretzels, and pasta.

Several studies have shown that chocolate milk provides "unique benefits" during the recovery period after strenuous exercise. Endurance athletes (not older adult strength trainers) who drank fat-free chocolate milk had elevated markers of muscle protein repair compared to those who drank carbohydrate beverages. Still, it may be helpful for older adults and you can consider adding to your recovery nutrition.

Calorie needs

Calories are fuel used for exercise. *NIH SeniorHealth* recommends the following calorie intake for women and men age 50 and older:

Women

- 1,600 calories a day if the level of physical activity is low (only performs activities associated with day-to-day life)
- 1,800 calories daily if moderately active (walks the equivalent of one to three miles a day at three to four miles p er hour)
- 2,000 to 2,200 calories if an active lifestyle (walks the equivalent of more than three miles a day at three to four miles per hour).

Men

- 2,000 to 2,200 calories a day if level of physical activity is low (only performs activities associated with typical day-to-day life)
- 2,200 to 2,400 calories daily if moderately active (walks the equivalent of one to three miles a day at three to four miles per hour)
- 2,400 to 2,800 calories if highly active (walks the equivalent of more than three miles a day at three to four miles per hour)

To determine the recommended intake of calories, grains, vegetables, fruits, dairy products, and protein based on your height and weight, go to the USDA's choosemyplate.gov and type My Daily Food Plan in the search engine. This can help you create an individual nutrition plan from which to begin.

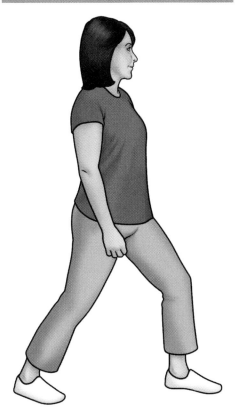

Take a long step forward with one foot, shift your weight forward, and keep the heel of your back foot in contact with the floor. Don't allow your front knee to extend beyond the front foot.

Preventing injuries

Exercise carries the risk of injury, but you can reduce the risks in several ways, beginning with warming up before a resistance training session and cooling down afterward.

Warming up

Regardless of the activity, every workout should begin with a warm up—the more prepared the body is, the less likely it is to get injured. But don't confuse warming up with stretching—whatever you do, don't stretch first. One sure way to strain a muscle or muscle group is to stretch it too far before doing any physical activity. A proper warm up for resistance training involved three stages:

Stage 1: Warm up to loosen up

Do something to slowly elevate your heart rate, increase circulation, raise the temperature of your muscles, and break a sweat. Wearing warm-up apparel while doing light physical activity is enough to increase the body temperature. Calisthenics, slow-paced swimming or cycling, and moderately paced walking or slow jogging can be effective first-stage warm ups.

Foam rollers are also a way to loosen muscle tissue. They involve applying pressure to the target area using the foam roller and changing the area of pressure by rolling back and forth along the length of the muscle. Foam rollers are inexpensive and can be an effective replacement for some of the stretches or massages normally performed in the second warm-up stage.

Stage 2: Static stretches

The second stage of a warm up is a little more complicated and a lot more controversial. Flexibility should be a part of every good warm up, according to the American College of Sports Medicine, but how to incorporate flexibility into the warm up is unclear.

Static stretches involve gently stretching a muscle or muscle group to a point of resistance and holding (but not bouncing) in that position for about 10 to 30 seconds. UCLA physical therapists recommend it for muscles known to be at risk of injury during certain activities, for muscles that have been previously injured, and for preventing diminished flexibility.

Stage 3: Dynamic stretches

Dynamic stretches move the body through a range of motion that mimics the activity that will follow. Dynamic stretches used to simply be called "warming up." Golfers and tennis players warm up by hitting shots they'll need on the course or court. Warming up for resistance training during stage two could be as simple going through the motions of exercises you will perform, but at slower speeds and with less resistance.

Ballistic stretching

The one kind of stretching to avoid is called ballistic. Ballistic stretches involve rapid, bouncing movement that moves the joint beyond its normal range of motion, or a range of motion limited by muscle tightness. Ballistic stretching can cause injury and soreness, and it doesn't allow enough time for the muscle tissues to adapt to the stretch. Instead of relaxing the muscle, it increases tension and makes it hard to stretch the surrounding connective tissues. Remember: no ballistic stretching and no bouncing.

Once you've completed the three warm-up stages—1) increased circulation/body temperature; 2) static stretching, if recommended by your physician or therapist; and 3) dynamic stretching—you are ready to begin your resistance training exercises.

Cooling down

You are not finished once your session ends. Take a few minutes to cool down. It reduces the risk of blood pooling in your legs, avoids the risk of a sudden drop in blood pressure, and allows your pulse rate to return to normal in a controlled manner.

A general guideline is to cool down until your pulse rate drops below 120 beats per minute, but that number does not take into consideration individual differences or age-related target heart rates. Your level of fitness improves as your recovery time declines. Here are some cool-down strategies:

Walk slowly for a few minutes after a session, or ride an exercise bike.Take a few minutes to go through some static stretches—the kind you do as part of your warm up. Static stretching increases subsequent range of motion. Include stretches for the upper body, core, and lower body.

See Box 2-13, "Lunges," Box 2-14, "Back extensions," and Box 2-15, "Overhead reach," for examples of cool-down static stretches.

BACK EXTENSIONS BOX 2-14

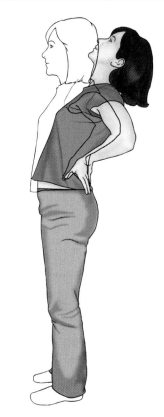

With your hands on the small of your back, slowly bend backward as far as comfortably possible.

OVERHEAD REACH BOX 2-15

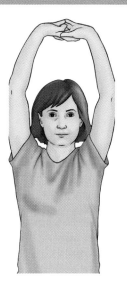

Extend your arms upward until you feel a stretch in your shoulders and upper back.

BOX 2-16

The shoulder is a common injury site in resistance training

An overview of documented shoulder injuries among older adults revealed that the shoulder complex—four joints and muscles that support them—was one of the most common areas injured during progressive resistance training. The shoulder is particularly susceptible to injury in exercises that place the arm extended above the head and behind the trunk. The review of studies also concluded that the best treatment for injury is prevention, including individualized programs, safe use of equipment, careful warm-up and cool-down periods, and correct range of motion.

Aging Clinical and Experimental Research, June 2014

BOX 2-17

Muscle scoreness
CAUSE
Unaccustomed exercise
TREATMENT
• Rest • OTC pain meds

BOX 2-18

Blisters
CAUSE
• Repetitive use irritation • Apparel/shoes that rub
TREATMENT
• Keep surface area intact • Skin torn: clean area • Skin missing: treat as abrasion • Apply dressing • Use doughnut pad over area

10 safety guidelines

The best way to lessen the risk of injury during resistance training is to use correct form. Specific technique instructions for 40 exercises are given in Chapter 3. Here are general safety tips:

1. Begin with a weight you can comfortably lift eight to 12 times to complete a set.
2. Choose lifts that involve the major muscle groups—arms, legs, chest, back, shoulders, and abdominals—but not all at the same time.
3. Move the weight in a smooth, controlled manner—don't rush or jerk the weights.
4. Maintain a grip that is firm, but not too tight.
5. Stop if you experience pain in your joints. However, expect general muscle soreness at first.
6. Maintain upright posture when the exercise allows it—back straight, head up, shoulders back.
7. Use muscle strength to move a weight, not momentum created by the weight itself.
8. Breathe out as you lift a weight; breathe in as you lower it. Avoid holding your breath at all times.
9. Work toward completing two to three sets with good technique before increasing the load.
10. Rest 48 hours between lifts involving the same muscle groups.

Common injuries

If you do get hurt during resistance training, some of the more common injuries are muscle soreness, blisters, strains, sprains, and cramps.

Older adults have a higher risk for many types of injuries, including those sustained while exercising, but there are ways to make strength training an injury-prevention strategy rather than an injury-risk factor. A 2014 study found that older adults are particularly susceptible to shoulder injuries (see Box 2-16, "The shoulder is a common injury site in resistance training"). Here is a look at other common injuries you may encounter:

Muscle soreness

Muscle soreness (see Box 2-17) is normal when beginning an exercise program and should resolve itself within a couple of days. Minimize it by warming up properly, gradually increasing exercise intensity and duration, and not overdoing it.

Delayed onset muscle soreness (DOMS) is also a condition

involving muscle overuse that usually develops a day or two after an especially hard workout. While some soreness after almost any vigorous exercise session is normal, DOMS is less common and probably indicates you have stressed the muscle tissues beyond their normal capacity.

The discomfort begins at a muscle-tendon junction and spreads throughout the affected muscle. DOMS lasts for a couple of days, but it's not a serious condition and the symptoms go away with rest.

Blisters

The most likely places for blisters (see Box 2-18) to develop for resistance-training exercisers are on the hands, but wearing gloves can reduce the risk.

Most blisters heal by themselves when the source of friction is removed. If the top area of the skin remains intact, a doughnut-like pad placed over the top protects the skin and relieves the discomfort. The fluid can be drained if you have access to a sterile needle, but the overlying skin should be left as a protective dressing.

If the skin has already been removed, treat the area as an abrasion. Wash it with mild soapy water or an antiseptic, then cover with a bandage, or ask about over-the-counter medicated blister dressings at a pharmacy. If the blister is not showing signs of healing within a few days, consult a physician.

Strains

Muscle strains (see Box 2-19) refer to stretched or torn muscles or tendons. They can occur almost anywhere, but especially the shoulders, neck, abdominal area, back, hip/groin, and legs. The injury often happens when a person needs to exert force with speed, but does not usually happen in strength training. It can be more of a problem with power training.

Strains are graded 1, 2, or 3 by physicians, according to the severity of the injury. Exercisers at higher risk for strained muscles are those who have a history of the injury, those who are overweight, and those in poor physical condition.

When the muscles are fatigued, overused, or not adequately warmed up, they are at increased risk of a strain. An imbalance between weak and strong muscles (hamstrings and quadriceps, for example) can also cause the injury, as can simply having an overly tight muscle group.

The initial treatment is rest with ice applications for 15 to 20

BOX 2-19

Strains

CAUSE
- Improper warm up or technique
- Sudden movement
- Overexertion
- Overuse
- Fatigue

TREATMENT
- Protection
- Rest
- Compression
- Ice
- Elevation
- OTC pain or anti-inflammatory meds

BOX 2-20

Sprains

CAUSE

Joint forced beyond normal range of motion

TREATMENT

- Protection
- Rest
- Ice first, heat later
- Compression
- Elevation
- Stabilization
- OTC pain or anti-inflammatory meds

minutes, three to four times a day for the first 48- to 72-hour period. After that, apply moist heat for the next 48- to 72-hour period, three to four times a day. If possible, use pillows to elevate the affected area during the first day and night.

Over-the-counter medications like aspirin, acetaminophen, ibuprofen, and naproxen may relieve pain. All but acetaminophen reduce both pain and inflammation. (Note that this may not be safe for older adults, so check with your doctor.)

Sprains

Although any joint can be sprained (see Box 2-20), the ankle is the most frequently injured part of the body among exercisers. The severity of the injury ranges from one that allows the person to return to normal activity in a few days to an injury that keeps a person out of action for several weeks. Those who have had a sprained ankle are the ones most likely to suffer the same injury again.

A sprained ankle is a stretch, tear, or rupture of at least one of the ligaments that hold the bones of the ankle joint together. The tears may be microscopic in size or large enough to represent a complete disruption of the fibers. One of the ligaments that wraps around the outside of the ankle is the weakest of the ankle ligaments, and is the one most frequently injured. It is possible that all three ligaments supporting the ankle, from front to back, may be sprained.

Symptoms vary according to the severity and grade—1, 2, or 3—of the sprain. The best-case scenario is mild pain, localized swelling, and tenderness, but no instability. You can walk, but don't try to jog or jump. Grade 2 and 3 sprains involve greater pain, a popping sound, bleeding, bruising, ankle instability, and difficulty in walking.

First aid is rest, ice, compression with an elastic bandage, wrap, or support device, elevation, and pain medication.

Some sprained ankles may be prevented by wearing protective shoes with side-to-side support, bracing or taping the ankle, and following the rule that says do not increase the resistance, frequency, or duration of an exercise by more than 10 percent a week.

Cramps

More than 90 percent of muscle cramps (see Box 2-21) happen in the hamstrings (back of the thighs), quadriceps (front of the thighs), or calves (back of the lower leg). The symptoms are unmistakable: sudden, involuntary, and painful muscle contractions.

Cramps can be caused by fatigue, hot and humid weather, prolonged overuse, dehydration, and electrolyte deficiencies. Electrolytes are potassium, calcium, and sodium, and people who take diuretics can develop electrolyte imbalances.

Attempts to relieve cramps include stretching the affected muscle group, applying pressure, and/or massage. A common mistake is trying to resume exercise immediately after the pain subsides. It won't work, and the muscle is likely to cramp again. If cramps persist, apply cold packs for 15 to 20 minutes, three to four times a day.

Reduce the risk of cramps returning by performing easy stretches and drinking plenty of fluids before, during, and after vigorous exercise.

Another way to help with cramps, as well as muscle soreness, is by using foam rollers over the problem area. These small cylinders of compressed foam are color coded according to firmness. White rollers are the softest, followed by blue or green (medium density), and black (firmest). White rollers are best for seniors and beginners, as they are the least dense and will allow some movement between the muscles, bones and the roller, and produce less pressure and pain.

Most foam rollers have a six-inch diameter with lengths ranging from 12 to 36 inches. A longer 36-inch roller is ideal for your back, as it will allow you to roll with it perpendicular to your back without worrying about slipping off the ends.

What's next?

The next chapter, *40 Strength & Power Exercises*, contains 40 total resistance-training exercises for the upper body, core, and lower body. Each exercise has a name, corresponding number for easy reference, instructions, and illustration.

BOX 2-21

Cramps

CAUSE
- Fatigue
- Prolonged overexertion
- Electrolyte depletion
- Dehydration

TREATMENT
- Stretch affected muscle
- Ice
- Pressure
- Massage
- Fluids

3 40 STRENGTH & POWER EXERCISES

The majority of exercises in this chapter require only your body weight or dumbbells, but included with those strength training methods are similar exercises that can be performed with equipment, such as stability balls, medicine balls, and resistance bands.

The exercises are organized from top to bottom—upper body first, then core, followed by lower body. The primary muscle or muscle group being exercised is noted before each exercise description.

Every exercise in this chapter can be modified to fit your fitness level and ability. Box 3-1, "Ways to modify resistance exercise programs," suggests specific ways.

What's next?

Chapter 4, *Strength and Power Programs*, contains 11 strength training packages—groups of exercises designed for entry level, intermediate, and advanced exercisers. A special section contains chair-based strength training exercises, and routines that involve only resistance bands, medicine balls, and stability balls.

BOX 3-1

Ways to modify resistance exercise programs

MODIFICATION	APPLICATION
Reduce the load	Begin with 3 pound dumbbells and work up to 8 pounds
Reduce the number of repetitions	Begin with 1-3 reps and work up to 8-10
Perform fewer sets	Begin with 1 set and work up to 2-3
Lower the intensity	Don't exercise to point of pain
Rest more between sessions	Take two days off between resistance training sessions
Manage time differently	Spread sessions throughout the day rather than all at once
Exercise muscles not affected	Upper body exercises if lower body is injured
Exercise larger muscles	Forearms, shoulders instead of wrists, fingers, hands
Change positions	Sit rather than stand while performing upper body exercises
Substitute type of training	Flexibility/balance instead of resistance
Modify the exercise	For instance, sitting instead of standing
Change equipment	Resistance bands rather than weights
Diversify exercises	More muscle groups rather than overworking a few
Use support devices	Knee braces, back supports, chairs, walls, benches

DUMBBELL ARM CURLS EXERCISE **1**
TARGET: BICEPS

- Standing or seated, hold a 3-5 pound dumbbell in each hand, arms down, palms out, and feet comfortably spread.
- Contract your abdominals and move the weights upward (together or alternately) by bending your elbows.
- Slowly lower the weights, stop, and repeat the movement.
- Work up to 8-10 repetitions, 2-3 sets.

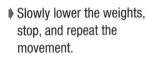

DUMBBELL HALF-KNEELING PRESSES
EXERCISE **2**

TARGET: SHOULDERS, BACK

- Place your right knee on the floor, with a cushion or pillow under it. Left leg bent.
- Left hand on left hip, hold a 1-5 pound dumbbell with your right hand, elbow bent so the dumbbell is at shoulder height.
- Extend your arm upward (without locking your elbow) and press the weight toward the ceiling.
- Hold for 1-2 second, then lower.
- Work up to 8-10 reps, 2-3 sets for each side.

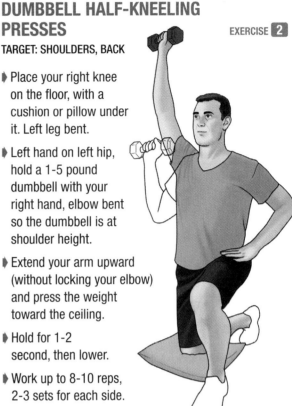

DUMBBELL OVERHEAD RAISES EXERCISE **3**
TARGET: SHOULDERS

- Seated or standing, hold a 3-5 pound dumbbell in each hand, elbows bent, weights at shoulder height.
- Slowly press lifts both weights toward the ceiling without locking your elbows.
- Hold for a second and slowly return to the starting position.
- Work up to 8-10 repetitions, 2-3 sets.

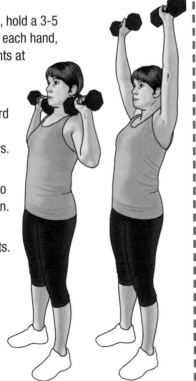

DUMBBELL LATERAL RAISES EXERCISE **4**
TARGET: SHOULDERS

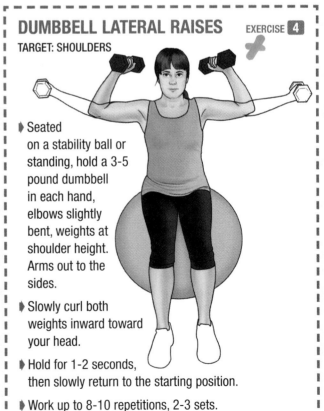

- Seated on a stability ball or standing, hold a 3-5 pound dumbbell in each hand, elbows slightly bent, weights at shoulder height. Arms out to the sides.
- Slowly curl both weights inward toward your head.
- Hold for 1-2 seconds, then slowly return to the starting position.
- Work up to 8-10 repetitions, 2-3 sets.

DUMBBELL FRONT RAISES

EXERCISE 5

TARGET: SHOULDERS

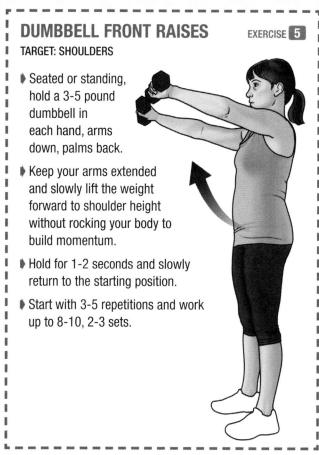

- Seated or standing, hold a 3-5 pound dumbbell in each hand, arms down, palms back.

- Keep your arms extended and slowly lift the weight forward to shoulder height without rocking your body to build momentum.

- Hold for 1-2 seconds and slowly return to the starting position.

- Start with 3-5 repetitions and work up to 8-10, 2-3 sets.

DUMBBELL SHRUGS

EXERCISE 6

TARGET: SHOULDERS

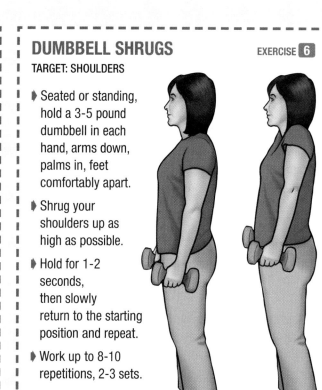

- Seated or standing, hold a 3-5 pound dumbbell in each hand, arms down, palms in, feet comfortably apart.

- Shrug your shoulders up as high as possible.

- Hold for 1-2 seconds, then slowly return to the starting position and repeat.

- Work up to 8-10 repetitions, 2-3 sets.

DUMBBELL TRICEPS KICKBACKS

EXERCISE 7

TARGET: TRICEPS

- Kneel with left knee bent and resting on a bench or bed, left arm supporting your body.

- Hold a 1-5 pound with right hand, arm at side, elbow bent 90 degrees.

- Extend your arm straight back, keeping your elbow close to your side.

- Work up to 8-10 reps for each arm, 2-3 sets.

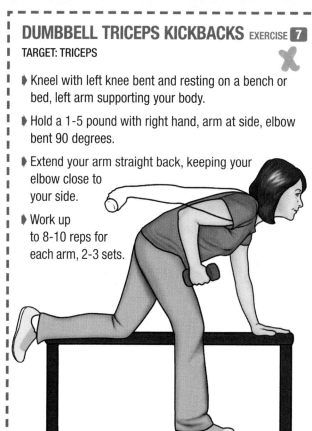

DUMBBELL UPRIGHT ROWS

EXERCISE 8

TARGET: SHOULDERS, BACK

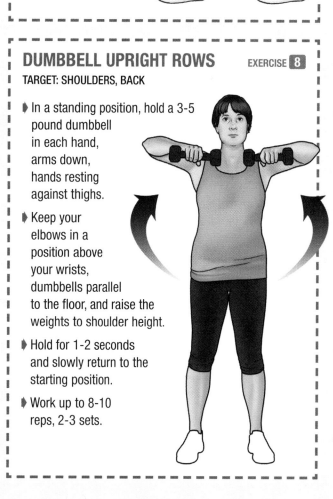

- In a standing position, hold a 3-5 pound dumbbell in each hand, arms down, hands resting against thighs.

- Keep your elbows in a position above your wrists, dumbbells parallel to the floor, and raise the weights to shoulder height.

- Hold for 1-2 seconds and slowly return to the starting position.

- Work up to 8-10 reps, 2-3 sets.

DUMBBELL UPPER BACK ROWS

EXERCISE **9**

TARGET: SHOULDERS, BACK

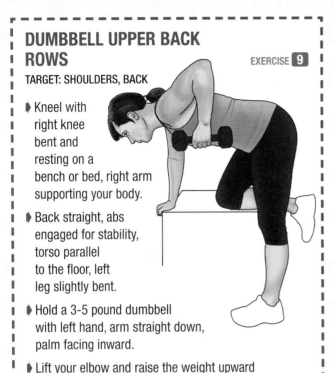

- Kneel with right knee bent and resting on a bench or bed, right arm supporting your body.

- Back straight, abs engaged for stability, torso parallel to the floor, left leg slightly bent.

- Hold a 3-5 pound dumbbell with left hand, arm straight down, palm facing inward.

- Lift your elbow and raise the weight upward toward your chest.

- Hold for 1-2 seconds and lower to the starting position.

- Work up to 8-10, 2-3 sets for each arm.

RESISTANCE BAND SEATED ROWS

EXERCISE **10**

TARGET: SHOULDERS, BACK

- In a seated position, legs stretched out, wrap a resistance band around your feet with arms extended.

- Hold one end of the band in each hand.

- Tighten your abs and pull the band toward your body.

- Hold for 2-3 seconds, work up to 8-10 times, 2-3 sets.

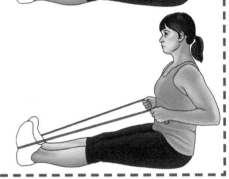

RESISTANCE BAND LAT PULL-DOWNS

EXERCISE **11**

TARGET: BACK

- Tie the middle of a resistance band around the top of door or other fixed object.

- Hold one end of the band in each hand, feet at hip width, knees slightly bent. Stand far enough away so your arms are extended overhead.

- Tighten your abs and pull the band down toward waist level.

- Hold for 2-3 seconds and slowly return to the starting position.

- Work up to 8-10 times, 2-3 sets.

RESISTANCE BAND STANDING CURLS

EXERCISE **12**

TARGET: BICEPS

- In a standing position, place your feet on the middle of a resistance band so that they anchor it on the floor.

- Hold the ends in both hands, arms down, palms facing forward, so that you feel a slight tension in the band.

- Tighten your stomach muscles and bend your elbows upward against the resistance of the band to a fully flexed position.

- Work up to 8-10 repetitions, 2-3 sets.

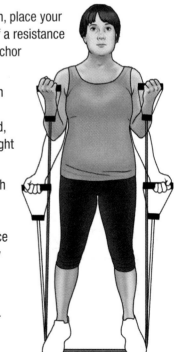

BACK STRENGTHENER

EXERCISE 13

TARGET: UPPER BACK

- Seated or standing, place your hands on their respective shoulders.

- Pull your shoulders back and squeeze your shoulder blades together until you feel the stretch.

- Hold for 1-2 seconds then release.

- Work up to 8-10 reps, 2-3 sets.

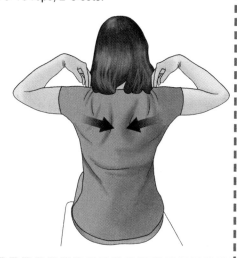

MODIFIED PUSH-UPS

EXERCISE 14

TARGET: ARMS, SHOULDERS

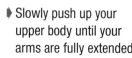

- Place your hands shoulder-width apart on the edge of a table, desk, or other sturdy object.

- Move your feet back so your body is at a 45-degree angle.

- Slowly push up your upper body until your arms are fully extended.

- Begin with 4-5 reps and work up to 8-10, 2-3 sets.

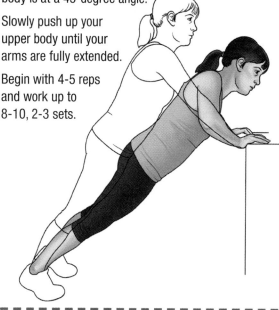

MEDICINE BALL EXCHANGE

EXERCISE 15

TARGET: ARMS, SHOULDERS, CORE

- Seated or standing, hold a 3-5 pound medicine ball in your right hand, elbow to your side, arm positioned outward.

- Raise the ball over your head and grasp it with the left hand.

- Switch the ball to your left hand and lower your arm until your elbow is at your side and your arm is positioned outward.

- Work up to 8-10 reps, 2-3 sets.

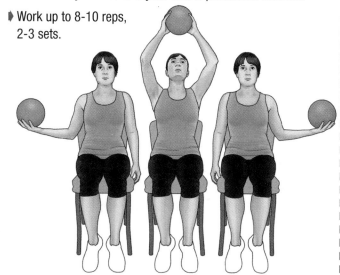

DUMBBELL FACE DOWN SHOULDER RAISE

EXERCISE 16

TARGET: SHOULDERS, ARMS

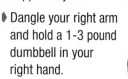

- Lie face down on a bench or similar support object.

- Dangle your right arm and hold a 1-3 pound dumbbell in your right hand.

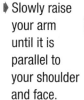

- Slowly raise your arm until it is parallel to your shoulder and face.

- Hold for 1-2 seconds and lower.

- Work up to 8-10 reps with each arm, 2-3 sets.

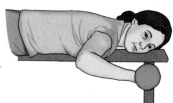

PLANKS

EXERCISE 17

TARGET: ABS, BACK, SHOULDERS

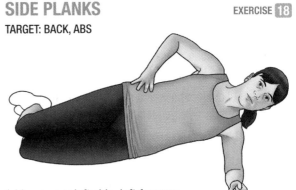

- Taking a position on the floor or mat, resting on your elbows and toes (or knees), head and neck in line with your body.
- Tighten your abs and position your body so that it forms a straight line.
- Work up to holding that position for 5-30 seconds.
- Rest and complete 2-3 sets.

SIDE PLANKS

EXERCISE 18

TARGET: BACK, ABS

- Lie on your left side, left forearm supporting your upper body and left side hips and legs touching the floor.
- Right hand on right hip.
- Contract your core muscles and lift your hips off the ground until your body is in a straight line.
- Hold for 5-10 seconds, relax, and return to the starting position.
- Work up to five repetitions on each side, 2-3 sets.

STABILITY BALL BACK EXTENSION

EXERCISE 19

TARGET: CORE, LOWER BACK

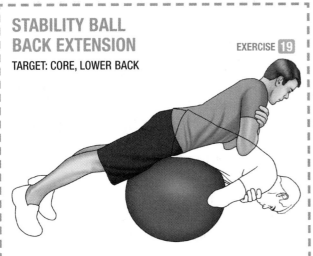

- Position your body so that your stomach and trunk are lying over a stability ball. Cross your arms over your chest.
- Lift your body until you form a straight line.
- Hold for 2-3 seconds then return to starting position.
- Work up to 8-10 repetitions, 2-3 sets.

STABILITY BALL BRIDGES

EXERCISE 20

TARGET: LOWER BACK

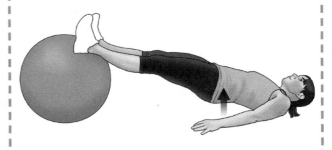

- Lie face-up on the floor, stomach tight, shoulders flat, and place your feet on a stability ball (or bench or couch).
- Tighten your buttocks and raise your hips to create a straight line with your body.
- Hold for 1-2 seconds, repeat for a total of 4-5 repetitions, and work up to 8-10.
- Begin with 1-2 sets and work up to 2-3.

MEDICINE BALL CRUNCH

EXERCISE 21

TARGET: CORE

- ◗ Lie on the floor, knees bent, holding a 3-5 pound medicine ball in both hands with arms extended upward.
- ◗ Slowly raise your torso until you feel your abs engaged then lower down.
- ◗ Work up to 8-10 reps, 2-3 sets.

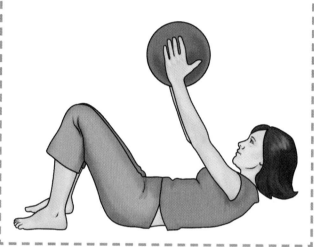

MEDICINE BALL OVERHEAD SLAMS

EXERCISE 22

TARGET: BACK, SHOULDERS, CORE

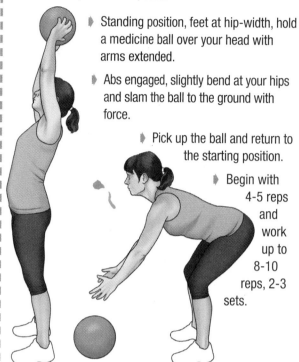

- ◗ Standing position, feet at hip-width, hold a medicine ball over your head with arms extended.
- ◗ Abs engaged, slightly bend at your hips and slam the ball to the ground with force.
- ◗ Pick up the ball and return to the starting position.
- ◗ Begin with 4-5 reps and work up to 8-10 reps, 2-3 sets.

MEDICINE BALL FIGURE 8s

EXERCISE 23

TARGET: BACK, CORE, SHOULDERS, ARMS

- ◗ Standing position, feet at hip width, hold a 3-5 pound medicine ball in front of your body, arms extended.
- ◗ Move the medicine ball in a side-to-side figure 8 motion to complete 1 repetition.
- ◗ Work up to 8-10 reps, 2-3 sets.

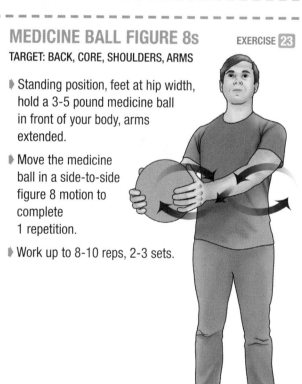

MEDICINE BALL CROSS-BODY SWINGS

EXERCISE 24

TARGET: CORE, BACK, SHOULDERS, ARMS.

- ◗ Standing or seated, hold a medicine ball with both hands in front of your body, arms extended.
- ◗ Move your arms alternately down and to the left, then up, across the front of your body, and up past your right shoulder.
- ◗ Move the ball back to the starting position and repeat the movement 8-10 times, 2-3 sets.
- ◗ Change starting positions and complete 8-10 reps, 2-3 sets on the opposite side.

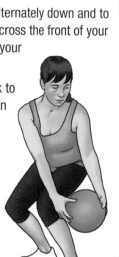
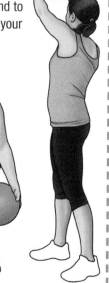

TRUNK RAISES
EXERCISE 25

TARGET: BUTTOCKS, HIPS, UPPER AND LOWER BACK

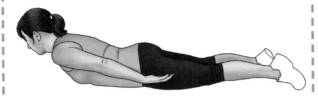

- Lie on your stomach, elbows bent, hands behind head.
- Without arching your neck, slowly lift your head and shoulders off the floor.
- Hold for 1-2 seconds, relax, and repeat five times, 2-3 sets.

MODIFIED SUPERMAN
EXERCISE 26

TARGET: BACK, CORE

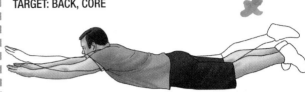

- Lie face down on a floor or mat, arms and legs extended forward.
- Tighten your buttocks and lift your legs, shoulders, and arms off the floor simultaneously.
- Flutter your hands and feet in an up and down motion for 2-3 seconds and slowly return to the starting position.
- Work up to 8-10 repetitions, 2-3 sets.

ALL-FOURS BACK EXTENSION
EXERCISE 27

TARGET: LOWER BACK, ABS

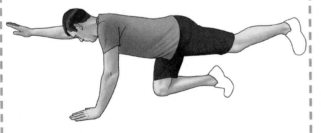

- Start from a hands and knees position on the floor.
- Slowly extend your right arm and left leg, hold for 2-3 seconds, then return to the starting position.
- Then slowly extend your left arm and right leg, holding for 2-3 seconds.
- Work up to 8-10 repetitions, 2-3 sets.

WINDSHIELD WIPERS
EXERCISE 28

TARGET: CORE

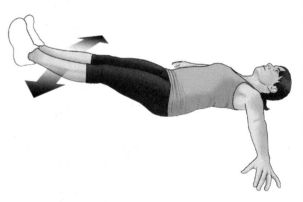

- Lie on your back, legs together and stretched out, arms extended at your sides.
- Contract the muscles of your abdomen and buttocks, lift your legs 6-12 inches off the ground and swing them to the left as far as they will go. Push your arms into the floor for support.
- Hold for a second and swing your legs to the right.
- Work up to 8-10 repetitions, 2-3 sets.

MEDICINE BALL SQUATS

EXERCISE 29

TARGET: BUTTOCKS, QUADS, HAMSTRINGS

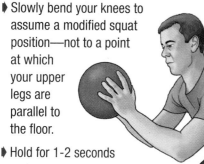

- Stand and hold a 3-5 pound medicine ball in front of you at chest level.

- Slowly bend your knees to assume a modified squat position—not to a point at which your upper legs are parallel to the floor.

- Hold for 1-2 seconds and slowly return to the starting position.

- Start with 1-5 repetitions and work up to 8-10 reps, 2-3 sets.

MEDICINE BALL OVERHEAD LUNGES

EXERCISE 30

TARGET: QUADS, BUTTOCKS, HAMSTRINGS

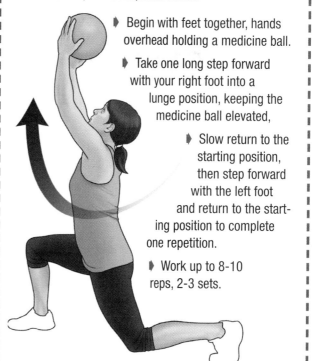

- Begin with feet together, hands overhead holding a medicine ball.

- Take one long step forward with your right foot into a lunge position, keeping the medicine ball elevated,

- Slow return to the starting position, then step forward with the left foot and return to the starting position to complete one repetition.

- Work up to 8-10 reps, 2-3 sets.

STABILITY BALL WALL SQUATS

EXERCISE 31

TARGET: BUTTOCKS, HAMSTRINGS, QUADS

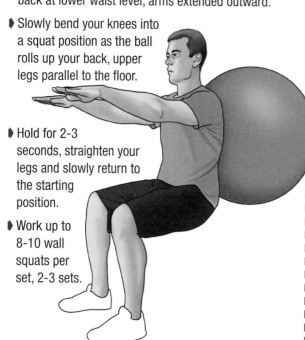

- In a standing position, place a stability ball behind your back at lower waist level, arms extended outward.

- Slowly bend your knees into a squat position as the ball rolls up your back, upper legs parallel to the floor.

- Hold for 2-3 seconds, straighten your legs and slowly return to the starting position.

- Work up to 8-10 wall squats per set, 2-3 sets.

RESISTANCE BAND SQUATS

EXERCISE 32

TARGET: BUTTOCKS, HAMSTRINGS, QUADS

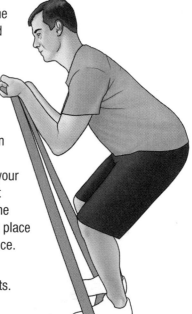

- Stand on the middle of a resistance band, legs hip-width apart.

- Hold one end of the band in each hand at chest level.

- Slowly lower your body into a semi-sitting position, as if sitting in a chair, then return to standing position, keeping your hands at the chest position, holding the resistance band in place to provide resistance.

- Work up to 8-10 repetitions, 2-3 sets.

SIDE LEG LIFTS

TARGET: THIGHS, HIPS, BUTTOCKS

EXERCISE 33

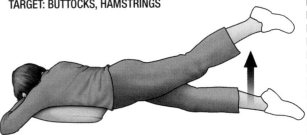

- Lie on left your side, right leg extended and on top of your left leg.
- Place your head on your left arm or on a cushion and place your right hand on the floor for balance.
- Slowly lift your right leg 12-18 inches off the floor and hold for 2-3 seconds.
- Slowly return to the starting position.
- Work up 8-10 repetitions and 2-3 sets.
- Change positions and perform the same exercise for the left leg.
- Add weight cuff around your ankles to increase the load.

PRONE STRAIGHT-LEG RAISES

TARGET: BUTTOCKS, HAMSTRINGS

EXERCISE 34

- Lie on your stomach with your abdomen and head supported.
- With knees straight, raise the left leg at the hip 2-3 feet.
- Do not arch your back or lift pelvis off the floor.
- Repeat the movement with the right leg.
- Work up to 8-10 repetitions for each leg, 2-3 sets.

ELEVATED LEG CIRCLES

TARGET: HIPS, THIGHS

EXERCISE 35

- Lie face-up on the floor or a mat, legs extended comfortably.
- Lift your left leg straight up as high as comfortable (bend your knees if needed).
- Move the left leg in circles 8-10 times, then stop and reverse directions for another 8-10 circles.
- Lower your leg and repeat with the right leg.
- Keep your abdominal muscles tight while performing leg circles, but don't hold your breath.
- Work up to 2-3 sets.

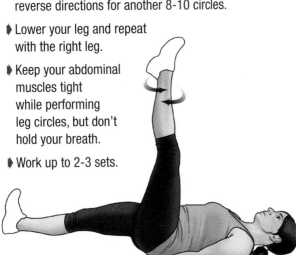

CLAMSHELLS

TARGET: HIPS, BUTTOCKS

EXERCISE 36

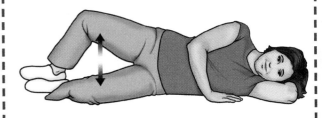

- Lie on your left side, right leg on top of the left, knees comfortably bent.
- Rotate the right leg up until your leg makes a 90-degree angle (or close to it) to the floor.
- Hold for a second and slowly return to the starting position.
- Work up to 8-10 repetitions, 2-3 sets.
- Change positions and complete the same number of repetitions and sets with the opposite leg.

DUMBBELL LUNGES

EXERCISE **37**

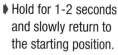

TARGET: QUADS, BUTTOCKS, HAMSTRINGS

▶ Hold a 3-5 pound dumbbell in each hand.

▶ Stand with feet at shoulder width, then take a giant step forward with your right leg and lower your body toward a position in which your upper right leg is parallel to the floor, left leg and knee almost touching the floor, back straight, head up.

▶ Hold for 1-2 seconds and slowly return to the starting position.

▶ Start with 4-5 repetitions and gradually work up to 8-10 reps, 2-3 sets for each leg.

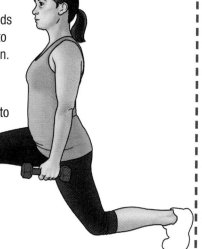

DUMBBELL SIDE LUNGES

EXERCISE **38**

TARGET: QUADS, BUTTOCKS, HAMSTRINGS

▶ Hold a 3-5 pound dumbbell in each hand, arms down or at sides, feet at shoulder width.

▶ Keep your right leg straight and take a big step to your left, bending your left knee.

▶ Back straight, head up.

▶ Plant your left foot, hold for 1-2 seconds, and return to the starting position.

▶ Start with 1-5 repetitions and gradually work up to 8-10, 2-3 sets for each side.

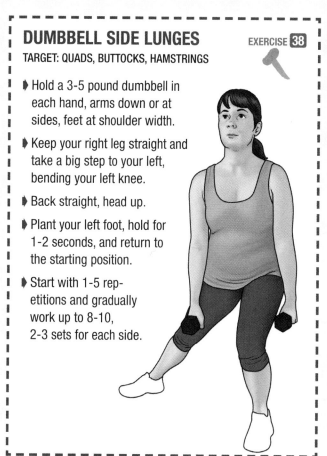

DUMBBELL STEP-UPS

EXERCISE **39**

TARGET: QUADS, HAMSTRINGS, HIPS

▶ Hold a 3-5 pound dumbbell in each hand, arms down, palms in

▶ Stand in front of the bottom step of a staircase (or a surface slightly higher, if stable)

▶ Step up with the left foot, then bring the right foot up and next to the left foot.

▶ Step down with the left foot first then the right foot.

▶ Repeat the sequence 8-10 times, 2-3 sets, leading each time with the left foot, then change the order and lead with the right.

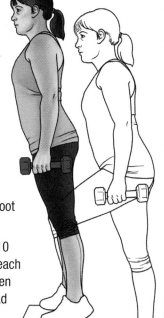

DUMBBELL CALF RAISES

EXERCISE **40**

TARGET: LOWER LEGS

▶ Hold a 3-5 pound dumbbell in each hand, arms down, palms in.

▶ Stand with your toes on a secure surface.

▶ Rise slowly on your toes while keeping your body straight.

▶ Hold for 1-2 seconds at the top of your movement, then slowly return to the starting position.

▶ Work up to 8-10 reps, 2-3 sets.

▶ Use heavier dumbbells to increase the load.

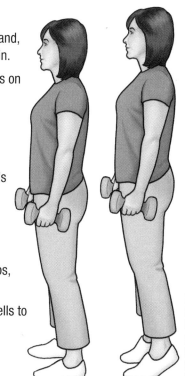

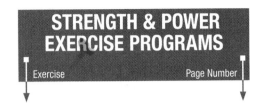
4 STRENGTH & POWER PROGRAMS

Choose exercises from the 40 described and illustrated in Chapter 3, or use one or more of the programs outlined in this chapter. The programs include routines based on using a single piece of equipment or prop, like a chair, medicine and stability ball, and resistance band. They are ideal for people with mobility issues and/or who enjoy exercises that do not require weights.

The other exercises are grouped into three levels: entry, intermediate, and advanced, and there are two different workouts for each category.

Mixing and matching the 40 exercises is okay, as long as you select exercises that strengthen all of the major muscle groups and body areas needed to improve strength and power.

The exercises also are color coded for easy identification—green for upper body, orange for core, and blue for lower body. By engaging (tightening) your abdominal muscles, many of the upper and lower body exercises can double as core exercises.

Guidelines

▶ **Number of days per week:** Two to three for each muscle group—upper body, core, and lower body.

▶ **Number of different exercises per session:** One to four for each group, but you can work on different areas of the body on different days—upper body on Mondays and Wednesdays, lower body on Tuesdays and Thursday, for example.

▶ **Amount of resistance or load:** A weight or other resistance you can lift, push, pull, or move eight to 12 times while using proper form. Begin with as little as one- to three-pound weights and gradually increase the load.

▶ **Order of strength training exercises when performed on the same day as other fitness exercises:** With flexibility training, flexibility first, strength training second. With balance training, the order doesn't matter—balance first, then strength training, or strength training first, then balance. With aerobic exercise plus strength training, it's more a matter of individual preference than exercise science. Some people prefer to begin with strength training, then do aerobic exercise. Others are more comfortable beginning with aerobic activities.

◗ **Increase exercise intensity, duration, or load:** No more than 10 percent per week.

◗ **Number of repetitions:** Begin with four to five for most lifts, fewer if necessary, but work up to eight to 10.

◗ **Number of sets:** Two to four, but adjust according to your age and physical condition.

◗ **Rest between sets:** The range is 30 seconds to five minutes, depending on the intensity, load, and number of sets. However, 30 seconds to one minute works for most of the exercises in these programs.

◗ **Rest between sessions:** 48 hours between exercises for the same muscle area.

◗ **Warm up:** A five- to 10-minute dynamic warm up that is challenging enough to break a sweat and increase circulation. Power walking and light calisthenics are typical warm-up activities.

◗ **Cool down:** Five to 10 minutes to cool off and lower the heart rate below 125 or 100 beats per minute (exercise literature is not consistent on an exact number, and the number varies from person to person). Walking and static stretches that mimic the movements you execute during a strength training session are ideal post-workout activities.

What's next?

Chapter 5, *The Strength & Power Workbook,* contains tools for scheduling and recording your strength and power training progress.

CHAIR-BASED EXERCISES #1

- ☑ **Dumbbell Arm Curls**
  - Exercise: **1**
  - Reps: 4-5 (work up to 8-10)
  - Sets: 1-2 (work up to 2-3)

- ☑ **Dumbbell Overhead Raises**
  - Exercise: **3**
  - Reps: 4-5 (work up to 8-10)
  - Sets: 1-2 (work up to 2-3)

- ☑ **Back Strengthener**
  - Exercise: **13**
  - Reps: 4-5 (work up to 8-10)
  - Sets: 1-2 (work up to 2-3)

- ☑ **Medicine Ball Exchange**
  - Exercise: **15**
  - Reps: 4-5 (work up to 8-10)
  - Sets: 1-2 (work up to 2-3)

CHAIR-BASED EXERCISES #2

- ☑ **Dumbbell Lateral Raises**
  - Exercise: **4**
  - Reps: 4-5 (work up to 8-10)
  - Sets: 1-2 (work up to 2-3)

- ☑ **Dumbbell Front Raises**
  - Exercise: **5**
  - Reps: 4-5 (work up to 8-10)
  - Sets: 1-2 (work up to 2-3)

- ☑ **Dumbbell Shrugs**
  - Exercise: **6**
  - Reps: 4-5 (work up to 8-10)
  - Sets: 1-2 (work up to 2-3)

- ☑ **Medicine Ball Figure 8s**
  - Exercise: **23**
  - Reps: 8-10
  - Sets: 1-2 (work up to 2-3)

RESISTANCE BAND EXERCISES

- ☑ **Resistance Band Standing Curls**
  - Exercise: **12**
  - Reps: 8-10
  - Sets: 2-4

- ☑ **Resistance Band Seated Rows**
  - Exercise: **10**
  - Reps: 8-10
  - Sets: 2-3

- ☑ **Resistance Band Lat Pull-Downs**
  - Exercise: **11**
  - Reps: 8-10
  - Sets: 2-3

- ☑ **Resistance Band Squats**
  - Exercise: **32**
  - Reps: 8-10
  - Sets: 2-3

STABILITY BALL EXERCISES

- ☑ **Dumbbell Lateral Raises**
  - Exercise: **4**
  - Reps: 4-5 (work up to 8-10)
  - Sets: 1-2 (work up to 2-3)

- ☑ **Stability Ball Back Extension**
  - Exercise: **19**
  - Reps: 1-5, then 8-10
  - Sets: 2-3

- ☑ **Stability Ball Bridges**
  - Exercise: **20**
  - Reps: 4-5 (work up to 8-10)
  - Sets: 1-2 (work up to 2-3)

- ☑ **Stability Ball Wall Squats**
  - Exercise: **31**
  - Reps: 8-10
  - Sets: 2-3

MEDICINE BALL EXERCISES

☑ **Medicine Ball Exchange**
- Exercise: `15`
- Reps: 4-5 (work up to 8-10)
- Sets: 1-2 (work up to 2-3)

☑ **Medicine Ball Overhead Slams**
- Exercise: `22`
- Reps: 8-10
- Sets: 2-3

☑ **Medicine Ball Cross-Body Swings**
- Exercise: `24`
- Reps: 8-10
- Sets: 2-3

☑ **Medicine Ball Crunch**
- Exercise: `21`
- Reps: 5-10
- Sets: 2-3

☑ **Medicine Ball Figure 8s**
- Exercise: `23`
- Reps: 8-10
- Sets: 2-3

☑ **Medicine Ball Overhead Lunges**
- Exercise: `30`
- Reps: 8-10
- Sets: 2-3

ENTRY LEVEL #1

☑ **Dumbbell Arm Curls**
- Exercise: `1`
- Reps: 4-5 (work up to 8-10)
- Sets: 1-2 (work up to 2-3)

☑ **Side Planks**
- Exercise: `18`
- Reps: 4-5 (work up to 8-10)
- Sets: 1

☑ **Clamshells**
- Exercise: `36`
- Reps: 4-5 (work up to 8-10)
- Sets: 2-3

☑ **Medicine Ball Exchange**
- Exercise: `15`
- Reps: 4-5 (work up to 8-10)
- Sets: 1-2 (work up to 2-3)

☑ **All-Fours Back Extension**
- Exercise: `27`
- Reps: 8-10
- 2-3 sets

☑ **Dumbbell Lunges**
- Exercise: `37`
- Reps: 4-5 (work up to 8-10)
- Sets: 2-3

ENTRY LEVEL #2

☑ **Dumbbell Lateral Raises**
- Exercise: `4`
- Reps: 4-5 (work up to 8-10)
- Sets: 1-2 (work up to 2-3)

☑ **Planks**
- Exercise: `17`
- Reps: 1 for 5-10 seconds
- Sets: 1-2, work up to 2-3

☑ **Side Leg Lifts**
- Exercise: `33`
- Reps: 4-5 (work up to 8-10)
- Sets: 1-2 (work up to 2-3)

☑ **Modified Push-ups**
- Exercise: `14`
- Reps: 4-5 (work up to 8-10)
- Sets: 1-2 (work up to 2-3)

☑ **Stability Ball Bridges**
- Exercise: `20`
- Reps: 4-5, (work up to 8-10)
- Sets: 1-2 (work up to 2-3)

☑ **Elevated Leg Circles**
- Exercise: `35`
- Reps: 4-5 (work up to 8-10)
- Sets: 1-2

INTERMEDIATE LEVEL #1

☑ **Dumbbell Arm Curls**
- Exercise: **1**
- Reps: 8-10
- Sets: 2-3

☑ **Dumbbell Lateral Raises**
- Exercise: **4**
- Reps: 8-10
- Sets: 2-3

☑ **Dumbbell Triceps Kickbacks**
- Exercise: **7**
- Reps: 8-10
- Sets: 2-3

☑ **Planks**
- Exercise: **17**
- Reps: 1 for 5-10 seconds
- Sets: 2-3

☑ **Stability Ball Bridges**
- Exercise: **20**
- Reps: 8-10
- Sets: 2-4

☑ **Modified Superman**
- Exercise: **26**
- Reps: 8-10
- Sets: 2-4

☑ **Side Leg Lifts**
- Exercise: **33**
- Reps: 8-10
- Sets: 2-3

☑ **Dumbbell Lunges**
- Exercise: **37**
- Reps: 4-5 (work up to 8-10)
- Sets: 2-3

☑ **Dumbbell Side Lunges**
- Exercise: **38**
- Reps: 8-10
- Sets: 2-3

INTERMEDIATE LEVEL #2

☑ **Dumbbell Half-Kneeling Presses**
- Exercise: **2**
- Reps: 8-10
- Sets: 2-3

☑ **Dumbbell Lateral Raises**
- Exercise: **4**
- Reps: 8-10
- Sets: 2-3

☑ **Dumbbell Front Raises**
- Exercise: **5**
- Reps: 8-10
- Sets: 2-3

☑ **Stability Ball Bridges**
- Exercise: **20**
- Reps: 8-10
- Sets: 2-4

☑ **Trunk Raises**
- Exercise: **25**
- Reps: 4-5
- Sets: 2-3

☑ **All-Fours Back Extension**
- Exercise: **27**
- Reps: 8-10
- Sets: 2-3

☑ **Side Leg Lifts**
- Exercise: **33**
- Reps: 8-10
- Sets: 2-3

☑ **Prone Straight-Leg Raises**
- Exercise: **34**
- Reps: 8-10
- Sets: 2-3

☑ **Dumbbell Side Lunges**
- Exercise: **38**
- Reps: 8-10
- Sets: 2-3

ADVANCED LEVEL #1

☑ **Dumbbell Half-Kneeling Overhead Presses**
- Exercise: **2**
- Reps: 8-12
- Sets: 2-4

☑ **Dumbbell Overhead Raises**
- Exercise: **3**
- Reps: 8-12
- Sets: 2-4

☑ **Dumbbell Lateral Raises**
- Exercise: **4**
- Reps: 8-10
- Sets: 2-4

☑ **Dumbbell Front Raises**
- Exercise: **5**
- Reps: 8-10
- Sets: 2-4

☑ **Planks**
- Exercise: **17**
- Reps: 1 for 5-10 seconds
- Sets: 2-3

☑ **Stability Ball Bridges**
- Exercise: **20**
- Reps: 8-10
- Sets: 2-4

☑ **Medicine Ball Overhead Slams**
- Exercise: **22**
- Reps: 8-10
- Sets: 2-3

☑ **Trunk Raises**
- Exercise: **25**
- Reps: 5
- Sets: 2-4

☑ **Resistance Band Squats**
- Exercise: **32**
- Reps: 8-10
- Sets: 2-3

☑ **Prone Straight-Leg Raises**
- Exercise: **34**
- Reps: 8-10
- Sets: 2-3

☑ **Elevated Leg Circles**
- Exercise: **35**
- Reps: 8-10 for each leg
- Sets: 2-4

☑ **Dumbbell Calf Raises**
- Exercise: **40**
- Reps: 8-10
- Sets: 2-4

ADVANCED LEVEL #2

☑ **Dumbbell Overhead Raises**
- Exercise: **3**
- Reps: 8-12
- Sets: 2-4

☑ **Dumbbell Front Raises**
- Exercise: **5**
- Reps: 8-10
- Sets: 2-3

☑ **Dumbbell Upright Rows**
- Exercise: **8**
- Reps: 8-12
- Sets: 2-4

☑ **Dumbbell Face Down Shoulder Raise**
- Exercise: **16**
- Reps: 8-12
- Sets: 2-4

☑ **Medicine Ball Crunch**
- Exercise: **21**
- Reps: 5-10
- Sets: 2-3

☑ **All-Fours Back Extension**
- Exercise: **22**
- Reps: 1 for 5-10 seconds
- Sets: 2-4

☑ **Modified Superman**
- Exercise: **26**
- Reps: 8-10
- Sets: 2-4

☑ **Windshield Wipers**
- Exercise: **28**
- Reps: 8-10
- Sets: 2-4

☑ **Medicine Ball Squats**
- Exercise: **29**
- Reps: 8-12
- Sets: 2-3

☑ **Side Leg Lifts**
- Exercise: **33**
- Reps: 8-10 for each leg
- Sets: 2-3

☑ **Dumbbell Step-Ups**
- Exercise: **39**
- Reps: 8-10
- Sets: 2-4

☑ **Dumbbell Calf Raises**
- Exercise: **40**
- Reps: 8-12
- Sets: 2-4

Action plan checklist ☑

- Make the decision to begin a resistance-training program. ☐

- Get medical clearance from your doctor. ☐

- Choose an exercise package or program. ☐

- Find comfortable and practical workout clothes and shoes. ☐

- Get the necessary equipment, if any, to perform your exercises. ☐

- Decide on a place where you live to do your exercises, or join a fitness center or gym. ☐

- Make a list of achievable first-week or first-month program goals (number of exercises, repetitions, or sets) ☐

- Schedule two to three non-consecutive exercise days for the first week. ☐

- Begin your program. ☐

- Keep records. ☐

5 THE STRENGTH & POWER WORKBOOK

The first step to beginning a resistance program is to have a plan, and Box 5-1, "Action Plan Checklist," is a 10-point planning tool to help you get into exercise mode.

In the rest of this chapter, you'll find the Daily Strength & Power Exercise Log to record the details of your daily workouts, and a Two-Week Workbook to manage your overall fitness and track your progress.

Daily strength & power exercise log

The Daily Strength & Power Exercise Log (see Box 5-2) can be copied and used to record the exercises, number of repetitions, and number of sets on a daily basis. An example of a typical day is provided, but enter the information that will best help you manage your workouts and stay motivated. Seeing a record of what you accomplish is a proven method of successfully participating in a program.

Two-week workbook

The Two-Week Workbook (see page 62) lets you manage your overall fitness to ensure you complement your strength and power training with workouts devoted to aerobics, balance, and/or flexibility. One week is filled out as a sample to follow. Make copies of the other weekly workbook and use it to create an ongoing history of your fitness.

BOX 5-2

DAILY STRENGTH & POWER EXERCISE LOG

DAY	EXERCISE NAME	NUMBER	REPS	SETS	NOTES
EXAMPLE	DB arm curls	1	10	2	START: 9:00am
	DB Presses	3	8	3	
	Semi sits	27	5	2	
	DB lunges	28	6	3	FINISH: 9:20am
MONDAY					
TUESDAY					
WEDNESDAY					
THURSDAY					
FRIDAY					
SATURDAY					
SUNDAY					

EASY EXERCISES WORKBOOK

EASY EXERCISES WORKBOOK

EXERCISE DAY OF THE WEEK	UPPER BODY EXERCISES (SEE PAGES 44-47)	CORE EXERCISES (SEE PAGES 48-50)	LOWER BODY EXERCISES (SEE PAGE 51-53)	☑ CHECK WHEN COMPLETED	COMMENTS
WEEK #1 MONDAY		✓*			*Notes
TUESDAY (CROSS-TRAINING)	Examples: aerobic class, treadmill workout, or yoga				*Notes
WEDNESDAY	✓*				*Notes
THURSDAY (CROSS-TRAINING)	Examples: aerobic class, treadmill workout, or yoga				*Notes
FRIDAY			✓*		*Notes
SATURDAY	REST				
SUNDAY	REST				

EXERCISE DAY OF THE WEEK	UPPER BODY EXERCISES (SEE PAGES 44-47)	CORE EXERCISES (SEE PAGES 48-50)	LOWER BODY EXERCISES (SEE PAGE 51-53)	☑ CHECK WHEN COMPLETED	COMMENTS
WEEK #2 MONDAY					
TUESDAY (CROSS-TRAINING)					
WEDNESDAY					
THURSDAY (CROSS-TRAINING)					
FRIDAY					
SATURDAY					
SUNDAY					

APPENDIX I: GLOSSARY

abdominals (abs): the muscles that support the area of the body between the chest and the pelvis

aerobic exercise: physical activity that increases the intake of oxygen and improves the cardiovascular and respiratory systems

atrophy: a decrease in the size of a muscle or muscle fiber

balance: the even distribution of weight that enables a person to remain upright and steady; also called equilibrium

ballistic stretching: a form of stretching that uses momentum to force a muscle group or joint beyond its normal range of motion

barbell: weight training equipment that has a long bar with weight on both ends

body composition: the fat mass percentage in a person's body compared to lean tissue

body mass index (BMI): a formula for categorizing weight in relation to height

body weight exercises: a type of exercise in which the weight of your body is used as resistance (example: modified push-ups)

closed grip: in weight lifting, a grip in which the fingers are wrapped around the bar of a dumbbell or barbell

cool down: exercise following a training session to allow the body to return to its normal state

core: the muscles of the hips, pelvis, trunk, shoulders, and neck

cramp: a sudden, involuntary, painful contraction of a muscle

cuff weights: weights with Velcro-type straps that wrap around wrists or ankles to provide resistance

delayed-onset muscle soreness (DOMS): a condition involving muscle overuse that usually develops a day or two after an especially hard workout

dumbbell: weight training equipment that has a short bar between two weighted ends

duration: the length of time an exercise session lasts

dynamic stretch: a stretch or exercise that involves movement

extension: straightening or extending a joint or limb of the body

flexion: bending a joint or limb of the body

flexibility: the range of motion through which a joint moves

foam roller: a cylinder-shaped exercise device made of dense foam that is used for self-massage or to loosen muscle tissue

free weights: dumbbells, barbells, or kettleballs (examples) used in resistance training

frequency: the number of strength training sessions conducted in a given period of time (2-3 times per week, for example)

functional fitness: strength and agility that helps people perform the basic activities of daily living

hamstring: a muscle or tendon behind the upper part of the legs

intensity: the amount of stress placed on the body by an exercise

isometric: a type of muscle contraction in which force is applied against an object that does not move

ligament: a tissue that connects bones or cartilages

load: the amount of resistance provided by a weight or object

medicine ball: a heavy, solid ball used in resistance training

mobility: the ability to move in one's environment with ease and without restriction

muscle imbalance: refers to opposite muscle groups (biceps/triceps, for example) that are not balanced in terms of strength

muscular endurance: the capacity of a muscle to do work over a period of time

myofascial release: a type of therapy used to ease soft muscle tissue stiffness and pain

neutral spine position: one in which there are natural curves of the cervical spine/neck, thoracic spine/mid back, and lumbar spine/lower back

obesity: a higher level of being overweight in relation to height, sometimes defined as being 20 percent over healthy weight

osteoarthritis (OA): a disease characterized by the degeneration of cartilage and the underlying bone

osteopenia: lower than normal bone density

osteoporosis: a disease in which the bones are weak, brittle, and porous

overhand grip: holding a dumbbell or barbell with the palms down

overweight: a weight that is unhealthy for a person of a given height

Pilates: an exercise program that consists of 25 to 50 low-impact strength and endurance movements to improve posture, balance, and flexibility

quadriceps (quads): large muscles on the upper front area of the legs

power: the ability to exert force against resistance with speed.

repetition (rep): a single act of lifting or moving a part of the body against resistance

repetition maximum (RM): the maximum amount of weight a person can lift at one time (in one repetition)

resistance bands: elastic bands that act as resistance against movement during resistance training

resistance training: a form of exercise that involves movement or attempted movement against resistance (or load)

sarcopenia: age-related loss of muscle mass and strength

set: the number of repetitions of an exercise movement

sprain: an injury caused by forcing a joint beyond its normal range of motion

stability ball: a large, inflatable ball used in various exercises

static stretch: stretching a muscle or muscle group to a point of resistance and holding the position

strain: a stretched or torn muscle or tendon, informally referred to as a pulled muscle

strength: the ability to exert force against resistance

strength training: exercises in which a person lifts or moves objects that create resistance in order to gain muscle strength or endurance

Superman: a floor exercise that strengthens muscle of the core

tai chi: a combination of relaxation, meditation, deep breathing, and slow, gentle, continuous, and structured movements

tendon: a tissue that connects muscles to bones and cartilage

30-second Chair Stand: a test used to measure leg strength and endurance

Timed Up and Go: a test that measures strength, power, balance, and agility

torso: the trunk of the body

underhand grip: holding a dumbbell or barbell with the palms up

volume: the total amount of weight lifted during an exercise session (number of repetitions times the number of sets)

warm up: exercise that prepares the body for more intense exercise

weight training: also called resistance training, in which a person lifts or moves weights in order to gain muscle strength or endurance

yoga: a type of exercise that incorporates movement, relaxation, and gentle breathing that may lead to improved balance, flexibility, range of motion, and strength

APPENDIX II: RESOURCES

American Academy of
Orthopaedic Surgeons
9400 West Higgins Road
Rosemont, IL 60018
847-823-7186
www.aaos.org

American Academy of Physical
Medicine & Rehabilitation
9700 West Bryn Mawr Avenue,
Suite 200
Rosemont, IL 60018-5701
847-737-6000
www.aapmr.org

American College of
Sports Medicine
401 West Michigan Street
Indianapolis, IN 46202-3233
317-637-9200
www.acsm.org

American Council on Exercise
4851 Paramount Drive
San Diego, CA 92123
888-825-3636
www.acefitness.org

American Heart Association
7272 Greenville Avenue
Dallas, TX 75231
800-242-8721
www.heart.org

American Orthopaedic Foot
& Ankle Society
9400 West Higgins Road
Suite 220
Rosemont, IL 60018
800-235-4855
www.aofas.org

American Physical
Therapy Association
1111 North Fairfax Street
Alexandria, VA 22314-1488
800-999-2782
www.apta.org/BalanceFalls/

American Podiatric
Medical Association
9312 Old Georgetown Road
Bethesda, MD 20814-1621
301-581-9200
www.apma.org

Arthritis Foundation
1330 W. Peachtree Street
Suite 100
Atlanta, GA 30309
404-872-7100
www.arthritis.org

Centers for Disease Control
and Prevention
1600 Clifton Road
Atlanta, GA 30329-4027
800-232-4636
www.cdc.gov

Center for Healthy Aging
c/o National Council on Aging
251 18th Street South
Arlington, VA 22202
202-479-1200
www.ncoa.org/improve-health/
center-for-healthy-aging

Department of
Rehabilitation Services
UCLA Health System
757 Westwood Plaza
Suite 3127
Los Angeles, CA 90094
310-825-5650
www.rehab.ucla.edu

National Association for
Health and Fitness
10 Kings Mill Court
Albany, NY 12205-3632
518-456-1058
www.physicalfitness.org

National Institute on Aging
31 Center Drive, MSC 2292
Bethesda, MD 20892
800-222-2225
www.nia.nih.gov

National Safety Council
1121 Spring Lake Drive
Itasca, IL 60143-3201
800-621-7615
www.nsc.org

National Strength &
Conditioning Association
1885 Bob Johnson Drive
Colorado Springs, CO 80906
719-632-6722
www.nsca.com

Office of Disease Prevention
and Health Promotion
U.S. Department of Health
and Human Services
1101 Wootton Parkway
Suite LL100
Rockville, MD 20852
email: odphpinfo@hhs.gov
www.health.gov

President's Council on Fitness,
Sports & Nutrition
1101 Wootton Parkway
Suite 560
Rockville, MD 20852
240-276-9567
www.fitness.gov

U.S. Department of Veterans Affairs
810 Vermont Avenue, NW
Washington, DC 20571
www.patientsafety.va.gov

YMCA of the USA
101 North Upper Wacker Drive,
Suite 1600
Chicago, IL 60606
800-872-9622
www.ymca.net